ADVANCES IN

Cardiac Surgery®

VOLUME 13

ADVANCES IN

Cardiac Surgery®

VOLUMES 1 THROUGH 9 AND VOLUME 11 (OUT OF PRINT)

ADVANCES IN

Cardiac Surgery®

VOLUME 13

Editor-in-Chief
Robert B. Karp, MD
Chief of Cardiac Surgery, University of Chicago, Chicago, Ill

Editorial Board
Hillel Laks, MD
Professor and Chief, Division of Cardiothoracic Surgery, University of
California Medical Center, Los Angeles, Calif

Bartley P. Griffith, MD
The Henry T. Bahnson Professor, University of Pittsburgh, Presbyterian
University Hospital, Pittsburgh, Pa

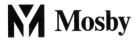 Mosby

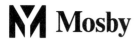 **Mosby**

Publisher: Cynthia Baudendistel
Developmental Editor: Jennifer Richardet
Manager, Periodical Editing: Kirk Swearingen
Production Editor: Amanda Maguire
Project Supervisor, Production: Joy Moore
Production Assistant: Betty Dockins

Printed in the United States of America
Printing/binding by The Maple-Vail Book Manufacturing Group

Editorial Office:
Mosby, Inc.
11830 Westline Industrial Drive
St. Louis, MO 63146

Customer service: periodical.service@mosby.com
              www.mosby.com/periodicals/

International Standard Serial Number: 0889-5074
International Standard Book Number: 0-8151-2719-7

Contributors

Sandy Abdelsayed
Manager, Clinical Affairs, MicroMed Technology, Inc, Houston, Tex

Robert Benkowski, BSME
Vice President, Engineering, MicroMed Technology, Inc, Houston, Tex

Stephen B. Colvin, MD
Associate Professor of Clinical Surgery, Chief, Division of Cardiothoracic Surgery, Department of Surgery, New York University School of Medicine, New York, NY

Kotturathu Mammen Cherian, MS, FRACS
Emeritus Professor in Cardiothoracic and Vascular Surgery, Tamil Nadu Dr. MGR. Medical University; Director, Institute of Cardiovascular Diseases, Madras Medical Mission, Chennai, India

B. Reddy Dandolu, MD
Resident, Cardiothoracic Surgery, MCP Hahnemann University School of Medicine, Philadelphia, Pa

Tirone E. David, MD
Professor of Surgery, University of Toronto; Chief, Division of Cardiovascular Surgery, Toronto General Hospital, Toronto, Ontario, Canada

Richard M. Engelman, MD
Professor of Surgery, University of Connecticut School of Medicine, Farmington, Conn; Clinical Professor of Cardiothoracic Surgery, Tufts University School of Medicine, Medford, Mass; and Chief, Cardiac Surgery, Baystate Medical Center,Springfield, Mass

Aubrey C. Galloway, MD
Professor of Surgery, Division of Cardiothoracic Surgery, Department of Surgery, New York University School of Medicine, New York, NY

Eugene A. Grossi, MD
Associate Professor of Surgery, Division of Cardiothoracic Surgery, Department of Surgery, New York University School of Medicine, New York, NY

Ziyad M. Hijazi, MD, MPH
Professor of Pediatrics and Medicine, Section of Pediatric Cardiology, Pritzker School of Medicine; Chief, Section of Pediatric Cardiology, University of Chicago Children's Hospital

Katherine Hillebrand
Research Assistant, Northwestern University Medical School, Evanston Hospital, Evanston, Ill

Suellen Irwin, RN
Research Associate, Michael E. DeBakey Department of Surgery, Baylor College of Medicine, Houston, Tex

Marshall L. Jacobs, MD
Chief, Section of Cardiothoracic Surgery, St. Christopher's Hospital for Children; Professor of Cardiothoracic Surgery, MCP Hahnemann University School of Medicine, Philadelphia, Pa

Angelo La Pietra, MD
Research Fellow in Cardiothoracic Surgery, Division of Cardiothoracic Surgery, Department of Surgery, New York University School of Medicine, New York, NY

Bryan E. Lynch, BSME, MBA
Director of Operations, MicroMed Technology, Inc, Houston, Tex

Deborah Morley, PhD
Vice President, Clinical Affairs, MicroMed Technology, Inc, Houston, Tex

Kona Samba Murthy, MCh
Senior Consultant, Institute of Cardiovascular Diseases, Madras Medical Mission, Chennai, India

George P. Noon, MD
Professor of Surgery, Michael E. DeBakey Department of Surgery; Chief, Division of Transplant and Assist Devices, Baylor College of Medicine; Executive Director, Multi-organ Transplant Center, The Methodist Hospital, Houston, Tex

Hermann Reichenspurner, MD, PhD
Associate Professor, Department of Cardiac Surgery, University Hospital Grosshadern, Ludwig-Maximilians-University, Munich; Director, Minimally Invasive Cardiac Surgical Program, University of Munich, Germany

Todd K. Rosengart, MD
Associate Professor of Surgery, Northwestern University Medical School;
Head, Division of Cardiothoracic Surgery, Evanston Northwestern
Healthcare, Evanston Hospital, Evanston, Ill

Edward D. Verrier, MD
Chief, Division of Cardiothoracic Surgery, University of Washington
Medical Center; William K. Edmark Professor of Cardiovascular Surgery;
Vice Chairman, Department of Surgery, University of Washington School
of Medicine, Seattle

David J. Waight, MD
Assistant Professor of Clinical Pediatrics, Section of Pediatric
Cardiology, Pritzker School of Medicine, University of Chicago
Children's Hospital

Contents

CHAPTER 1

Port-Access Surgery: Pros and Cons

Hermann Reichenspurner, MD, PhD
Associate Professor, Department of Cardiac Surgery, University Hospital Grosshadern, Ludwig-Maximilians-University, Munich; Director, Minimally Invasive Cardiac Surgical Program, University of Munich, Germany

The advent of minimally invasive surgery was brought about primarily by a desire to minimize the trauma incurred by patients who undergo cardiac operations. The port-access method developed by Stevens et al[1] was designed to alleviate the distress of coronary surgery in two ways: (1) by offering an extracorporeal cardiopulmonary bypass system, thereby preserving the myocardium, and (2) by reducing the length of the incision. Beyond minimizing incision length, Port-Access technology (Heartport, Inc, Redwood City, Calif) allows for single- and multivessel coronary artery bypass grafting (CABG) and mitral valve repair or replacement (MVR) to be undertaken through port-incisions or a minithoracotomy.

The essence of the Port-Access system lies in the component design of the endoluminal cardiopulmonary bypass (Endo-CPB; Heartport) system. The Endo-CPB system, developed in conjunction with Stanford University, comprises 5 main components: (1) a Y-shaped femoral arterial return cannula or direct aortic cannula, (2) a femoral venous cannula for the drainage of the right atrium, (3) an endopulmonary vent catheter for venting, (4) an endoaortic balloon occlusion catheter (endoaortic clamp) for aortic occlusion, root venting, and the application of antegrade cardioplegia, and (5) an endocoronary sinus catheter for application of retrograde cardioplegia (Fig 1). This system allows for the use of a regular cardiopulmonary bypass system, including a venting and cardioplegic cannula, without the necessity to open the chest.

The preferred methods for observing the position and movements of the various cannula and catheters comprising and sup-

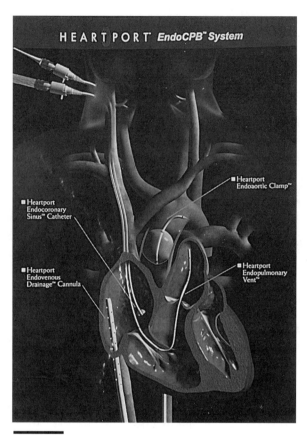

FIGURE 1.

Port-Access-Endo-Cardiopulmonary Bypass System (Courtesy from Heartport Inc, Redwood City, Calif)

porting the Endo-CPB are transesophageal echocardiography (TEE) and fluoroscopic imaging. Particular modes of observation and tracking have been developed in conjunction with the application of the Port-Access technology, and these will be discussed at length below. The application of the Endo-CPB system, together with CABG, MVR, or atrial septal defect surgery being undertaken through small incisions, is called "Port-Access" surgery.

Although the Port-Access surgical procedure has been extended to feature prominently in the performance of MVR and has recently been applied to perform atrial septal defect closure, it was originally developed for the purpose of CABG. Indeed, more than half (57%) of all Port-Access procedures are for CABG; thus, a brief elucidation of the Port-Access CABG method is offered.

CORONARY ARTERY BYPASS GRAFTING

The Port-Access CABG technique involves the performance of coronary artery surgery through a small thoracic access and employs the above-mentioned endovascular bypass system for the provision of extracorporeal circulation and cardioplegic arrest. Femoral arterial or direct aortic and femoral venous access are used for installation of CPB, and aortic occlusion, root venting, and antegrade cardioplegia are all performed with use of an endoaortic clamp (Heartport), a transfemoral or transaortic endoaortic occlusion catheter.

The Port-Access system was initially developed and tested at the Stanford University School of Medicine, and the University of Dresden began a clinical program based on the performance of Port-Access CABG in March 1996.[2,3] In this initial study, 42 patients with lesions of the left anterior descending coronary artery underwent Port-Access CABG. After the University of Dresden study was completed, a similar clinical trial was conducted at the University of Munich; in the Munich study, the Port-Access CABG method was used to treat 12 cases of single-vessel coronary artery disease and 5 cases of multivessel disease. In the following passage, the 2 clinical studies are described as one, since they were performed by the same surgeons.

PATIENTS AND METHODS

Of the 45 male and 14 female patients, the median age was 58 ± 12.5 years, the eldest being 78 and the youngest 31. The median preoperative left ventricular ejection fraction was 0.65 ± 0.2, and it ranged from a low of 0.35 to a high of 0.78. All patients were afflicted with angina pectoris and qualified as CCS stage 2 or 3.

Patients were first submitted for preoperative assessment of the abdominal aorta and the iliac and femoral arteries by Doppler sonography. The ascending and descending aorta were evaluated by means of TEE to screen for atherosclerotic disease of the aorta and major aortic valve incompetence.

After the administration of anesthesia, a double-lumen endotracheal tube was placed to ventilate the right lung. The right internal jugular vein was punctured by using a 9F introduction system for later insertion of the endopulmonary vent catheter. Invasive blood pressure was monitored through the right and the left radial arteries, echocardiographic observation of the surgical process in its entirety was enabled through use of a TEE probe.

The patients were placed in a supine position such that the left shoulder was elevated and fixed at about 30°. The draping and preparation of the patients ensured that the entire chest and both groins were left visible and easily accessible in the event that the procedure was converted to a conventional CABG with a median sternotomy.

The Port-Access CABG procedure involved making a small left anterior thoracic incision of approximately 5 to 8 cm (median of 7.5 cm) parasternally above the fourth intercostal space. The left internal mammary artery was directly dissected distally down to below the sixth rib and proximally up to the first rib. This process involved the preparation, ligation, and division of all the major side branches.

Meanwhile, as the left internal mammary artery was being prepared, the femoral vessels were dissected through a small incision made above the right groin and surrounded in umbilical tape. The Y-shaped femoral arterial return cannula was then placed into the femoral artery. The correct placement of the arterial cannula was achieved through use of a long guide wire, measuring approximately 100 mm. After these initial arterial preparations, the 28F venous cannula was inserted into the femoral vein and positioned into the right atrium using TEE control.

A guide wire was once again used to set the endoaortic clamp in place and was entered through the second opening of the Y-shaped arterial cannula. Fluoroscopy and TEE control were used to monitor the immersion of the guide wire and the occlusion catheter into the descending, and then into the ascending, aorta. Recently, an alternative direct aortic cannula has become available; it is placed through a thoracic port penetrating the second intercostal space and into the ascending aorta.

CPB was begun after the correct placement of the endoaortic clamp. Venous drainage was augmented by a centrifugal pump connected to the heart-lung machine.

An incision was made in the pericardium just above the left anterior descending artery (LAD), extending above the ascending aorta. Pericardial stitches were made to the left and to the right of the ascending aorta, and adhered to the skin incision so as to render the ascending aorta visible and enable it to be pulled toward the skin incision.

In the cases of multivessel Port-Access CABG, the proximal anastomoses of the vein grafts were performed first by using a side-biting clamp to the ascending aorta (Fig 2).

The balloon of the endoaortic clamp was then inflated, with use of diluted radiocontrast agent. The balloon was placed approximately 2 cm above the aortic valve; the right radial artery pressure

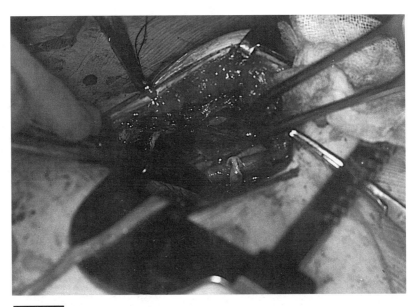

FIGURE 2.
Port-Access-CABG: Proximal bypass anastomosis of a saphenous vein graft to the ascending aorta through the mini-thoracotomy.

was monitored intensely, in an effort to prevent the occlusion of the bracheocephalic trunk. On complete inflation of the balloon, both its pressure and the aortic root pressure were carefully monitored. Cardioplegic solution could finally be administered through the proximal end of the endoaortic clamp and cardoplegic arrest attained. Further root-venting could be performed through the distal end of the endoaortic catheter.

The coronary arteries were then dissected, and the distal vein anastomoses were performed. The use of gauzes aided in rendering the coronary arteries visible. The left internal mammary artery to LAD artery anastomoses was the last to be completed, whereupon the balloon was deflated and cardiac reperfusion was started. After the bypass grafts were de-aired and full hemodynamic stability was achieved, CPB was discontinued. Finally, the chest and groin incisions were sealed after decannulation, and surgical drainage was performed by using 1 chest tube.

RESULTS
The combined results of the initial clinical experiences with Port-Access CABG at the University of Dresden and the University of Munich are as follows. In total, 58 of 59 patients (98.3%) survived

and proceeded to make acceptable recoveries: there were 3 major complications. One retrograde aortic dissection occurred, which led to the death of a patient 5 days after surgery. Preoperatively, this patient had displayed evidence of peripheral vascular disease. Moreover, this patient was treated with the first generation of endoaortic clamps: since the introduction of the second generation of endoaortic clamps in October 1996, no further aortic dissection has been documented in this study. The second major complication was derived from the dissection of 1 iliac artery. The third complication arose because the removal of the femoral arterial cannula necessitated the reconstruction of the femoral artery with use of a patch. All other complications observed were minor: These consisted of 3 pleural effusions, 3 small wound infections, 3 cases of postoperative hemorrhage, and 2 cases of lymphatic fistula in the groin. One patient had transient hemiparesis for 24 hours, likely derived from an air embolism, yet went on to make a complete recovery.

Postoperative angiography indicated patent anastomoses in 98% of the patients (1 graft was occluded). Altogether, 3 patients displayed signs of diffuse stenotic LAD artery disease (at the site of anastomosis in 1 patient and distally to the site of anastomosis in 2 others). These were treated successfully with subsequent percutaneous transluminal coronary angioplasty.

In summation, the clinical experience of the universities of Dresden and Munich with the performance of 59 Port-Access CABG surgeries yielded an anastomotic patency of 98% and a mortality rate of 1.7%.

In the clinical experience with CABG at New York University, largely the same procedure was applied in the performance of CABG using the Port-Access system.[4] The average patient age was 59.8 years, ranging from 34 to 82. Thirty-seven patients were afflicted with multivessel coronary artery disease and thus received multivessel CABG, while 16 underwent single-vessel CABG surgery.

There were no operative deaths and no perioperative myocardial infarctions, neurological deficits, or conversions to sternotomy. Reoperation was necessitated by hemorrhage in 4 patients; a pulmonary embolism occurred in 1 patient. Moreover, the occlusion of a right coronary artery graft in 2 patients necessitated the performance of angioplasty.

However, as shown in the angiograms procured for 42 of the 49 patients (86%), left internal mammary artery grafts were 100% patent, while a patency rate of 96% was exhibited for all grafts overall.

In 1999, the results of a "prospective multicenter study on Port-Access coronary artery bypass grafting" were published by Grossi et al,[5] compiling the results of the Port-Access CABG experiences of 3 institutions. From October 1996 to June 1998, 302 patients underwent CABG by means of the Port-Access method: 76 underwent single grafts (25.2%), 110 underwent double (36.4%), 73 (24.2%) triple, and 43 (14.2%) quadruple. The average age of patients was 60.7 years. The results of the study were then compared with The Society of Thoracic Surgeons (STS) Database records for regular CABG procedures. The results of the prospective multicenter study yielded a total (30-day) hospital morbidity rate of 0.99, which was comparable to that predicted by the STS data (1.2%). Perioperative transmural myocardial infarction was 0% (vs 1.3%) and ventilatory support for more than 1 day was 1.7% (vs 3.8%). Higher rates than that foreseen by the STS database were found for reoperation for bleeding (3.3% vs 1.9%) and stroke (1.7% vs 1.2%).

CONCLUSION

From the Dresden-Munich clinical experiences, as well as from those at New York University and the multicenter study, it seems that the main advantages gained in CABG from using the Port-Access system are as follows. Because of the use of CPB and cardioplegic arrest, all coronary arteries can be adequately accessed for revascularization through a small anterior thoracotomy, and thus the anastomoses can be performed on the arrested heart, allowing for a safe anastomosis. In addition, the same incision can be used for the performance of proximal bypass anastomoses. Moreover, patient trauma is reduced, and thus recovery time is shortened. This raises the morale of patients. On the other hand, times of surgery are significantly prolonged, or costs are increased. There remains a risk of arterial injury and dissection and a slightly increased incidence of postoperative bleeding and stroke necessitating reintervention.

MITRAL VALVE REPAIR AND REPLACEMENT

Approximately 27% of all Port-Access operations concern the mitral valve. Port-Access mitral valve replacement or repair (PA-MVR) is undertaken through a small right mini-thoracotomy by using the same endovascular CPB system (as opposed to the traditional entrance through a median sternotomy). The system uses femoral arterial or direct aortic and femoral venous access for CPB and the same endoaortic occlusion catheter for aortic occlusion and application of antegrade cardioplegia. It makes use of the technique originally developed for minimally invasive coronary artery surgery, but modified for mitral valve surgery. The first applications of the Port-Access technique to human beings undergoing mitral valve surgery were commenced in 1996 at the universities of Stanford, Dresden, and Leipzig.

The standard procedure for the performance of Port-Access mitral valve repair and replacement (PA-MVR) surgery has been updated in recent years. Today, most of these procedures include the assistance of 2- or 3-dimensional video screening and robotics. In this method, direct visualization of the mitral valve is achieved; in addition, a thorascope is inserted and this projects a 2- or 3-dimensional videoscopic image of the mitral valve on a screen. In some cases, the AESOP robotic arm (Computer Motion Inc, Goleta, Calif) has been used in conjunction with the videoscope system, holding the camera with greater stability. The AESOP system also allows for voice-controlled movement of the camera. These aids have been deemed necessary for the creation of precise anterior and lateral mini-thoracotomies, approximately 4 to 5 cm in length.

The following documents the clinical experiences of the University Hospital Munich in performing such video- and robot-assisted PA-MVR.[6]

PATIENTS AND METHODS

Fifty patients, 26 male and 24 female, with a median age of 61.5 years (range, 36-77) underwent PA-MVR. Thirty-six patients had mitral valve insufficiency, and 14 had combined mitral valve disease. In total, 26 patients underwent MVR for quadrangular resection of the posterior leaflet and the placement of an anuloplasty ring and 3 underwent repair of the anterior leaflet. Twenty-four patients required valve replacement in which a mechanical or biological valve prosthesis was substituted for the natural valve. All patients were monitored through a 3-dimensional endoscopic camera system (VISTA; Cardiothoracic Systems Inc, Westborough, Mass), and the final 20 were monitored with the additional aid of the AESOP robotic arm.

Preoperatively, all patients underwent assessment of the abdominal aortic, iliac and femoral arteries with use of Doppler sonography. Evidence of a major peripheral vascular disease served as a contraindication for the use of the endovascular CPB system. Moreover, TEE screening of all patients was undertaken to assess the mitral valve disease and to evaluate the condition of the ascending and descending aorta. The TEE also served to eliminate cases of moderate or major aortic valve incompetence.

After the induction of anesthesia, a double-lumen endotracheal tube was placed to allow left lung ventilation. The right internal jugular vein was punctured by using a 9F introduction system, for later insertion of the endopulmonary vent catheter. The left and the right radial arteries were used for invasive blood pressure monitoring to detect partial or total occlusion of the brachio-cephalic trunk by the endoaortic balloon. Finally, the insertion of the endopulmonary vent catheter was placed by the anesthesiologist through the right internal jugular vein over a balloon-tipped pulmonary artery catheter, using pressure control and, when necessary, fluoroscopy.

The patient was placed in a supine position with the right shoulder being elevated about 30°. The right arm was attached to the body dorsally to the posterior axillary line. The patient was prepared and draped in such way that the whole right side of the chest was accessible—as well as the whole sternum, in case the operation had to be converted to a conventional procedure with sternotomy. Moreover, both groins were prepared for surgical access in the event of an abortion of the Port-Access procedure and the need to switch to other methods.

At surgery, a small (4- to 7-cm) right submammary incision was performed, and the fourth intercostal space was entered, after left single-lung ventilation. The pericardium was opened about 2 cm anterior and parallel to the right phrenic nerve from the superior vena cava, and the incision was extended down to the origin of the inferior vena cava. Silk sutures were used to secure the anterior pericardium to the skin margins; the posterior pericardium was pulled through the skin dorsally to the thoracic incision. These sutures also helped to retract the diaphragm from the surgical view. A soft tissue retractor (Heartport) was used to open the intercostal space and retract the subcutaneous tissue and underlying musculature. In parallel, the right femoral artery and vein were dissected and encircled by using umbilical tapes. A 15-mm thoracic port was inserted posterior to and cranially of the thoracic incision, enabling the insertion of the 3-dimensional endoscopic camera. Before insertion, the camera had been secured to a firm camera holder. This holder was then attached to the voice-controlled robotic arm to provide stable camera guidance. The entire setup is pictured in Figs 3 and 4.

After heparinization, arteriotomy was performed and the Y-shaped femoral arterial return cannula (sizes, 23F in 43 patients and 21F in 7 patients) was placed into the femoral artery. Alternatively, a direct aortic cannula can be placed through a tho-

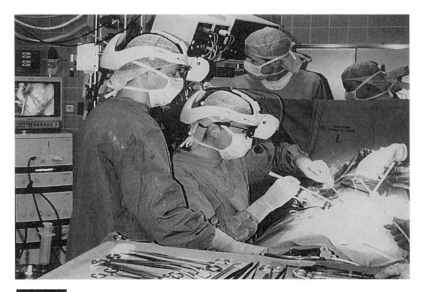

FIGURE 3.
Intraoperative set-up during a Port-Access mitral valve repair. The surgeon sits on the right side of the patient operating through the mini-thoracotomy with shafted instruments. The surgeon operates using a combination of direct visualization together with the endoscopic image presented in the head-mounted display.

racic port penetrating the second intercostal space into the ascending aorta. Then, a purse-string suture was done on top of the femoral vein, and a 28F venous cannula was inserted into the femoral vein and positioned into the right atrium by using TEE guidance. Before the initiation of CPB, the endoaortic clamp was positioned by using a guidewire through the other opening of the Y-shaped arterial cannula. If no resistance was felt during the insertion of the guidewire, the endoaortic clamp was forwarded into the ascending aorta by means of TEE control only. In case of any slight resistance, fluoroscopy was used to guide the wire and the endoaortic clamp into the ascending aorta. This occurred in 12 patients. In 3 patients, the left groin had to be used for arterial cannulation because of atherosclerotic disease of the right femoral artery.

Venous drainage was augmented by means of a centrifugal pump connected to the heart-lung machine. After initiation of CPB, the heart was electrically fibrillated to allow for correct placement of the endoaortic balloon, which was inflated about 2 cm above the aortic valve as monitored by TEE (see Fig 1). During this process, right radial artery pressure was carefully monitored to detect the ovoid occlusion of the bracheocephalic trunk by the endoaortic balloon. After the balloon was fully inflated, balloon and aortic root pressures were monitored continuously. A balloon pressure above 300 mm Hg was usually associated with complete occlusion of the aorta. Any residual flow past the balloon was monitored and detected with Doppler TEE. After full occlusion, antegrade cardioplegic solution was administered.

The left atrium was incised above the origin of the right upper pulmonary vein as done in regular mitral valve surgery. The incision was extended by using endoscopic scissors cranially and caudally. A holder for the left atrial retractor was inserted parasternally through a 5-mm thoracic port and inside the chest connected to a left atrial retractor (Heartport). The 3-dimensional camera was inserted and positioned in the chest in such a way that the whole

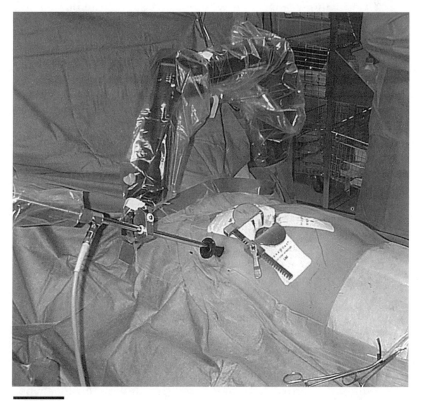

FIGURE 4.
Port-Access-mitral valve repair: mini-thoracotomy and set-up of the AESOP-robotic arm holding a 3-D-endoscope.

mitral valve apparatus was visible on the screen. An additional soft suction device was inserted through a small additional port incision, which was later used for chest drain insertion. This suction device was inserted into the left atrium. The mitral valve was then carefully assessed and evaluated with regard to potential reconstructive surgery. The camera-holding robotic arm was guided by voice control. The microphone was attached to a head-mounted display, which allowed a 3-dimensional videoscopic image. In case of a posterior mitral valve prolapse, a quadrangular resection was done followed by readaption of the posterior anulus and continuous suture of the leaflet tissue. The valve was then tested for competence. In case of additional anular dilatation a full mitral valve ring was measured and implanted by an interrupted or continuous 2-0 suture. If no annular dilatation was detected, a posterior ring (Cosgrove ring; Baxter GmbH, Unterschleissheim, Germany) was inserted with use of a 3.0 continuous monofilament suture. Thereafter, the valve was again tested for competence. In 3 cases with an anterior valve prolapse a chordal plasty was done with a pledged Gore-Tex suture, attaching the anterior leaflet back to the papillary muscle in 1 patient and chordal shortening in 2 cases.

In case of mitral valve replacement, the anterior leaflet was removed first and the posterior leaflet was kept in place. The valve was then measured and replaced with a mechanical or biological valve prothesis with use of interrupted annular valve sutures.

After the procedure a left ventricular vent catheter was inserted through the valve and the left atrium was closed with a running 3-0 monofilament suture. Before the suture was tied, careful retrograde deaeration was done through the atrium with use of the vent catheter. In addition, the ascending aorta was punctured with a small needle proximally to the inflated balloon. After complete deaeration, the balloon was deflated and reperfusion of the heart was started. Ventricular and atrial pacing wires were inserted, and after adequate reperfusion patients were weaned from CPB and the femoral cannulas were removed. All patients had intraoperative TEE control to assess the result of mitral valve repair and to detect any paravalvular leak after valve replacement. After hemostasis was obtained, 1 chest tube was inserted and the thoracic and femoral incisions were closed.

The total operative time, duration of CPB and duration of cardioplegic arrest were monitored. In addition, all major postoperative factors, such as the length of intensive care unit (ICU) stay and total hospital stay, were recorded. Follow-up studies were conducted by means of physical examination, 12-lead electrocardiography, transthoracic echocardiography (TTE), as well as by the procurement of a chest x-ray film 2 days after the surgery and again just before discharge. The first 40 patients underwent even more stringent follow-up sessions, including laboratory testing, 12-lead electrocardiography, a chest x-ray film, and TTE 12 weeks after surgery.

RESULTS

Of 52 patients, all but 2 underwent PA-MVR successfully. The 2 who did not were afflicted with major pleural adhesions and were consequently converted to standard mitral valve procedures. However, in the 50 that did undergo PAMVR, all procedures were largely uneventful, with no major complications and no aortic or arterial injury. Of those minor complications that did occur, 6% were in the groin and 6% were postoperative hemorrhaging, largely because of injury of intercostal vessels that necessitated operative revision. A postcardiotomy syndrome developed in 1 patient, and another had a right ventricular perforation, likely caused by the endopulmonary vent catheter. This complication was managed through the mini-thoracotomy.

The results were compared with those of 49 conventional mitral valve surgery cases undertaken during the same period. Although no significant differences were seen, there was a trend toward a longer duration of CPB and aortic crossclamp time in the PA-MVR group, however stay in the ICU and the duration of the total hospital stay were less in this group.

These results are consistent with the fact that 92% of patients had minor or no complaints of postoperative pain, and the remaining 8% complained only of moderate pain—all suggesting a diminished level of patient trauma.

Follow-up at 3 months was complete in 40 patients (80%). At this follow-up, most patients (85%) were in New York Heart Association (NYHA) class I, and no patient was in an NYHA class above 3. Transthoracic echocardiography revealed 1 minor paravalvular leak after replacement. One patient with grade 3 mitral insufficiency after the repair underwent subsequent reoperation and conventional valve replacement. Follow-up was completely uneventful for 38 patients (95%). Mortality was 0% and prevalence of reoperation was 2% among all patients operated on.

From the clinical experience, the University of Munich group concluded that anterior mini-thoracotomies are the preferred incisions for conducting minimally invasive mitral valve repair and replacement surgery. These anterior mini-thoracotomies are less traumatic to the patient and result in scars that are asthetically preferable. Videoscopic surgery was deemed necessary for minimizing the length of surgical incisions; by virtue of presenting a clear view of the surgical field, and the provision of better depth perception through the 3-dimensional exposure, the procedure could be undertaken with greater precision. Moreover, videoscopic vision provided a great method for the adequate inspection of the incision and the thoracic ports before closure. Finally, it was generally agreed that the trauma of surgery was minimized, despite the increased duration of the procedure compared with conventional procedures.

A different technique uses the same mini-thoracotomy access, the so-called micro–mitral valve operation described by Chitwood.[7] In his series, the author also emphasizes the necessity for video assistance to allow for accurate exposure of the mitral valve through the limited access. The only difference in his surgical technique lies in the fact that direct transthoracic aortic cross-clamping was applied by using a specifically designed transthoracic aortic clamp. This technique seems to be equally safe; there is a potential danger of pulmonary artery injury in direct transthoracic clamping as compared with the potential danger of retrograde aortic dissection with use of the endoaortic balloon occlusion catheter. Apart from this technical difference, the results in the series published by Chitwood are excellent and compare favorably with conventional mitral valve surgery and some centers' results with PA-MVR.

In another series, published by Loulmet et al,[8] different surgical methods were compared for less-invasive mitral valve surgery. Twelve patients who underwent a mini-thoracotomy were compared with 10 patients who were operated on through a mini-sternotomy. The series consisted of 19 mitral valve repairs and 2 replacements. In 2 cases it was necessary to convert to a larger incision. Mortality was 0%, and the patients were discharged with normal valve function comparing the mini-thoracotomy and mini-sternotomy the authors were in favor of the small sternotomy approach for better exposure of the valve.

As a potential disadvantage, the parasternal or mini-sternotomy approach may require division of the left atrial roof and interatrial septum with possible postoperative arrhythmias. The mini-thoracotomy allows for the well-known entry through the interatrial groove into the left atrium and a direct access to the mitral valve.

A clinical study compiled by Vanermen et al[9] examined the results of 75 Port-Access mitral valve operations performed from February 1997 to November 1998. In total, 41 patients underwent mitral valve repair and 33 underwent mitral valve replacement with the assistance of video screening and shafted instruments. The average age of the patients was 59.3 years (range, 32-83 years). The majority of the patients fell under NYHA functional class II; 45 had myxoid degeneration, 21 rheumatic disease, 4 chronic endocarditis, 2 annular dilatation, and 2 sclerotic disease, 1 from myxoma and 1 a paravalvular leak after valve replacement.

Of the 75 patients, only 1 died, a day after operation as a result of a failed repair. One patient required immediate converison to sternotomy for treatment of a dissected aorta. Five patients required revision for treatment of postoperative bleeding. There were no cerebrovascular accidents due to thromboembolic phenomena and no paravalvular leakages owing to myocardial infarction.

The average length of stay in the ICU was approximately 2.5 days, and the average hospital stay came to about 9 days. The group noted a striking discrepancy in the length of ICU stay between the first 30 patients operated on, and the last 38, which was attributed to greater familiarity with the system.

It was concluded from the results that the Port-Access method of undertaking mitral valve repair and replacement is acceptably safe and holds the advantage of being less painful for the patient. In this experience too, hospital and ICU stay were found to be shortened by the minimal trauma of this method, especially once greater familiarization with the Port-Access method was obtained. Video-assisted visualization was noted for its benefit not only during the actual process of mitral valve repair and replacement, but also toward the finale of the procedure, serving to investigate the quality of repair of valve leaflets and the strength of closures. There remains, however, a certain risk of retrograde aortic dissection.

Another study of video-assisted Port-Access mitral valve surgery was undertaken by Mohr et al.[10] In this study, 129 patients were treated by the Port-Access method, dating from June 1996 to December 1998. The 67 patients treated from June 1997 to December 1998 were treated with voice-controlled robotic assistance, eliminating the need for an extra assistant (group II). The first 62 underwent the Port-Access method with standard 3-dimensional video-assistance (group I). Seventy-two patients underwent mitral valve repair, and 57 underwent mitral valve replacement. All patients were treated through a 4-cm lateral mini-thoracotomy by using femoro-femoral bypass and endoaortic clamping, which was monitored by means of TEE and transcranial Doppler techniques.

Most of the serious complications occurred in group I. In total, 3 patients afflicted with acute retrograde aortic dissection (2 in group I and 1 in group II) and 1 patient who experienced injury of the left ventricular posterior wall were converted to a standard sternotomy procedure. Two patients from group I underwent a mini-sternotomy to replace an unstable endoaortic clamp. Six patients experienced serious hemorrhaging and had to undergo reexploration. Moreover, group I faced a greater prevalence of neurologic complications.

Hospital mortality was relatively high for the first 62 patients: the mortality rate for group I was 11.3% within a follow-up period of 804 ± 35 days, compared with 3.0% for group II, with a follow-up period of 568 ± 12 days.

In group II (those whose procedures were assisted by the voice-controlled robotic arm), although CPB time was not significantly reduced, the length of the surgical process in its entirety was greatly reduced. The robotic camera-holding arm enabled surgeons to better concentrate on tissue manipulation by providing a stable, non-varying view of the tissue. Moreover, the lens of the robotic arm–controlled camera required significantly less intermittant cleaning than did a hand-held camera. Furthermore, the ability to zoom in and out on a subject of vision was a boon to the ability to repair. Nevertheless, the overall mortality rate was still high in the total series, but it was significantly less in group II.

ATRIAL SEPTAL DEFECT CLOSURE

Although most current applications of Port-Access surgery have been in the fields of CABG and mitral valve repair and replacement, Port-Access technology has also proved to be an effective method for minimally invasive closure of atrial septal defects.

Median sternotomy has been the traditional method for artial septal defect closure. However, surgeons at several centers have advocated the use of the right thoracotomy instead of the more traumatic sternotomy. Yet the use of the right thoracotomy as the access point has 2 significant drawbacks: (1) it is difficult to insert the aortic cannula in patients with deep chest diameters, and (2) the incision made for the thoracotomy is rarely less than 10 to 12 cm in length. Thus, using Port-Access technology as a means of performing minimally invasive atrial septal defect surgery has been investigated.

A report compiled at the University Hospital Grosshadern in Munich describes the use of the Port-Access surgical method for the minimally invasive closure of an atrial septal defect in 7 patients with an ostium secundum defect.[11] First, a preoperative Doppler sonography screening of the pelvic and femoral arteries served as a precaution against potential retrograde aortic dissection. Then, with use of the femoral endovascular bypass system, a Port-Access atrial septal defect closure was performed. The process was undertaken through a 3- to 5-cm right submammarian mini-thoracotomy with videoscopic and robotic assistance. In addition, the insertion of a superior vena cava cannula into the right internal jugular vein was the only diversion from the standard Port-Access mitral valve surgical technique. The heart was arrested throughout the surgical procedure by virtue of an endoaortic balloon catheter, which, beyond aortic occlusion, also served for the provision of antegrade cardioplegic solution. Moreover, careful retrograde and antegrade deaeration was undertaken as a precaution against the development of air embolisms.

The defect closures were performed without any complications, and the mini-thoracotomy and videoscopic image were found sufficient for adequate access to the atrial septal defect and, more generally, the right atrium. The trauma of surgery was thus minimized, to the extent the patients were released from the hospital 4 or 5 days after the procedure.

From the case study, it was concluded that Port-Access technology was well suited to provide minimally invasive atrial septal defect closure leading to an excellent cosmetic result (Fig 5).

PROS

Port-Access surgery allows a surgeon to perform cardiac surgery on the arrested heart, using CPB, through limited or even endoscopic incisions. The CPB system can be inserted by a femoral or a direct aortic approach, and all additional catheters can be placed intraluminally. Currently, the Port-Access system is the only available and proven bypass system that allows for endoscopic cardiac surgery to be performed on the arrested heart. Several hundred Port-Access CABG procedures and Port-Access mitral valve surgeries have been reported on, operations performed through skin incisions only 3 to 5 cm in length. With careful patient selection and proper operative management, the overall results are satisfactory and the recovery of patients seems to be accelerated when compared with patients who are conventionally operated on.

CONS

Because of the different placement and monitoring techniques, the insertion and use of such a system requires adequate training and leads to increased operation times, at least during the first series of

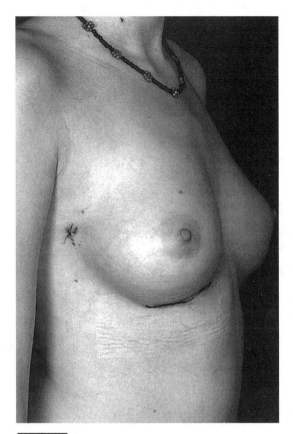

FIGURE 5.
Cosmetic result after Port-Access-ASD closure.

cases. The use of all catheters and cannulas can be cumbersome in some cases, and operating room schedules must be flexible.* Patients undergoing Port-Access surgery should be carefully selected and screened for evidence of peripheral or aortic vascular disease. A number of aortic dissections have been documented in the past; however, in recent series the incidence of such dissections is less than 1%.[5]

At least in cases operated on through mini-thoracotomies, the use of a transthoracic clamp is a potential well-accepted and less costly alternative to the use of an endoaortic balloon catheter.

---

* The costs for the Port-Access Endo-CPB system are markedly increased when compared with conventional CPB.

ACKNOWLEDGEMENT

The author wishes to thank Ms. Sarah Shennib for her help in preparing the manuscript.

REFERENCES

1. Stevens JH, Burdon TA, Peters WS, et al: Port-Access coronary artery bypass grafting: a proposed surgical method. *J Thorac Cardiovasc Surg* 111:567-573, 1996.
2. St Goar FG, Siegel LC, Stevens JH, et al: Catheter based cardioplegic arrest facilitates Port-Access cardiac surgery. *Circulation* S I94:52, 1996.
3. Reichenspurner H, Gulielmos V, Wunderlich J, Dangel M, Wagner FM, Pompili MF, et al: Port-Access coronary artery bypass grafting with the use of cardiopulmonary bypass and cardioplegic arrest. *Ann Thorac Surg* 65:413-19, 1998.
4. Shwartz DS, Ribakove GH, Grossi EA, Schwartz JD, Buttenheim PM, Baumann FG, et al: Single and multivessel port-access coronary artery bypass grafting with cardioplegic arrest: Technique and reproducibility. *J Thorac Cardiovasc Surg* 114:46-52, 1997.
5. Grossi EA, Groh MA, Lefrak EA, Ribakove GH, Albus RA, Galloway AC, et al: Results of a prospective multicenter study on port-access coronary bypass grafting. *Ann Thorac Surg* 68:1475-1477, 1999.
6. Reichenspurner H, Boehm DH, Gulbins H, Schulze C, Wildhirt S, Welz A, et al: Three-dimensional video and robot-assisted port-access mitral valve operation. *Ann Thorac Surg* 9:1176-1182, 2000.
7. Chitwood WR Jr, Wixon CL, Elbeery JR, Moran JF, Chapman WHH, Lust RM, et al: Video-assisted minimally invasive mitral valve surgery. *J Thorac Cardiovasc Surg* 114:773-782, 1997.
8. Loulmet DF, Carpentier A, Cho PW, et al: Less invasive techniques for mitral valve surgery. *J Thorac Cardiovasc Surg* 115:772-779, 1998.
9. Vanermen H, Wellens F, DeGeest R, Degrieck I, Van Praet F: Video-assisted Port-Access mitral valve surgery: from debut to routine surgery. Will Trocar-Port-Access cardiac surgery ultimately lead to robotic cardiac surgery? *Semin Thorac Cardiovasc Surg* 11:223-234, 1999.
10. Mohr FW, Onnasch JF, Falk V, Walther T, Diegeler A, Krakor R, et al: The evolution of minimally invasive mitral valve surgery—2-year experience. *Eur J Cardiothorac Surg* 15:233-239, 1999.
11. Reichenspurner H, Boehm DH, Welz A, Schulze C, Zwissler B, Reichart B. 3D-video- and robot-assisted minimally invasive ASD closure using the Port-Access technique. *Heart Surg Forum* 1: 104-106, 1998.

CHAPTER 2

Recent Advances in Reconstructive Surgical Management of Hypoplastic Left Heart Syndrome

B. Reddy Dandolu, MD
Resident, Cardiothoracic Surgery, MCP Hahnemann University School of Medicine, Philadelphia, Pa

Marshall L. Jacobs, MD
Chief, Section of Cardiothoracic Surgery, St. Christopher's Hospital for Children; Professor of Cardiothoracic Surgery, MCP Hahnemann University School of Medicine, Philadelphia, Pa

Lev et al[1] in 1952 described a complex he named "hypoplasia of the aortic tract," and subsequently Noonan and Nadas[2] coined the term "hypoplastic left heart syndrome" (HLHS) to include the entities of aortic stenosis or atresia with mitral stenosis or atresia along with a hypoplastic left ventricle and aorta. This entity does not include aortic atresia seen in patients with single left ventricle, complete transposition with tricuspid atresia, or mitral atresia and corrected transposition.[3]

A 1998 multi-institutional study by the Congenital Heart Surgeons Society[4] identified a variety of cardiac anomalies associated with aortic atresia in 323 neonates during a 4-year period. The most common was bilateral superior vena cava (28 cases), followed by intact atrial septum (13 cases), anomalous origin of the right subclavian artery from the descending thoracic aorta (11 cases), left ventricle to coronary artery fistula (8 cases), partial anomalous pulmonary venous connection (9 cases), total anomalous pulmonary venous connection (3 cases), single coronary orifice (4 cases), and pulmonary valve stenosis (3 cases). Among the noncardiac anomalies found in association with this complex were Turner syndrome (7 cases), microencephaly (3 cases), and tracheal esophageal fistula (2 cases). Reis et al[5] reported extracardiac anomalies to occur in 12% of their series. They also noted a very high incidence (53%) of associated anomalies among infants born prematurely. Turner syndrome again was the most common in their series, with the second most common being vertebral anomalies. Rychik et al[6] reported 18 cases of HLHS with intact atrial septum out of a total of 316 infants seen during a 6.5-year period, for an incidence of 5.7%. They identified 3 types of abnormal atrial septal morphology. First was a large left atrium with a thick prominent septum secundum and a thin septum primum adherent (type A, n = 12), second was a small left atrium with a thick muscular atrial septum (type B, n = 4), and last was a giant left atrium with a thin atrial septum with severe mitral regurgitation (type C, n = 2). Histopathology showed severely dilated lymphatics and arterialization of the pulmonary veins in the type with the severe degree of obstruction to left atrial egress (type B). Type A had the best prognosis, with 6 early survivors, although 3 of them died during the second stage. Overall, the outcome for infants born with HLHS and intact atrial septum is probably less satisfactory than for HLHS in general.

DIAGNOSIS AND PREOPERATIVE MANAGEMENT

Prenatal diagnosis of HLHS is established by means of fetal echocardiography. Chang et al[7] reported their experience with 22 consecutive cases diagnosed prenatally between 1986 and 1990. Postnatal echocardiography confirmed the diagnosis in all of these cases except one. They proposed that in utero transport of the fetus with suspected critical left ventricular outflow obstruction to a neonatal cardiac surgical center can result in improved neonatal condition and may improve overall survival. In a retrospective review of the obstetric management of 219 infants with HLHS, Reis et al[5] noted that most infants (74%) were delivered vaginally, and cesarian delivery was performed only for routine obstetric indications. In this population, the prenatal diagnosis was made in 37% of cases at a mean gestational age of 27 weeks. Karyotype analysis was performed in this group in 32 cases (15%). Chorionic villous sampling for chromosomal analysis could be done as early as 11 weeks of pregnancy. Once the diagnosis of HLHS is made based on fetal echocardiography, it is recommended that delivery be planned in proximity to a cardiac center experienced in treating children with this condition. This will not only be economical as compared with transporting a neonate who might require advanced support including ventilation, but also simplifies overall neonatal management and surgical planning.

Neonates with HLHS diagnosed postnatally may be hemodynamically stable but may be initially seen with a state of acidosis and hypoperfusion, and the definitive diagnosis is often not made until after multiorgan system failure is established. In such cases, the mainstays of therapy include institution of a prostaglandin infusion to reopen the ductus arteriosus, mechanical ventilatory support with the goal of achieving arterial blood gas values that result in a satisfactory balance of pulmonary and systemic blood flow, and supportive management until restoration of satisfactory perfusion results in improvement of end organ function. This may include the use of antibiotics, intravenous nutrition, and the judicious use of inotropic agents. In other instances, the postnatal diagnosis of HLHS may be established with echocardiography in the newborn nursery, based on suspicion of a cardiac disorder that is raised because of tachypnea, mild hypoperfusion, presence of a murmur, or arterial desaturation. In these instances, resuscitation is rarely necessary. Infusion of prostaglandin is begun, and the babies are transported to a cardiac surgical center. Most often this can be accomplished with the neonates breathing spontaneously, or with minimal ventilatory support on the lowest fraction of inspired oxygen (FIO_2) that provides adequate oxygenation. Reliable venous access for prostaglandin infusion is important to establish and maintain patency of the ductus arteriosus. A detailed postnatal echocardiogram is performed to define cardiac morphology. A variety of mechanisms have been used to address excessive pulmonary blood flow in the preoperative period. Some investigators favor the use of a hypoxic air mixture achieved by addition of nitrogen. Others favor the addition of carbon dioxide to the inspired gases, to increase the pulmonary vascular resistance and effect a more favorable balance of pulmonary and systemic blood flow.

In those cases where there is evidence of pulmonary venous obstruction, a restrictive interatrial communication may need to be enlarged. This may be accomplished in the cardiac catheterization laboratory by blade or balloon septostomy. Alternatively, these patients may be taken to surgery emergently, with the first procedure being either stage 1 palliation, or simple atrial septectomy (followed by stage 1 palliation several days later). Atz et al[8] reported on the management of 21 neonates with the diagnosis of HLHS with pulmonary venous hypertension who were taken to cardiac catheterization. They recommended performing either surgical atrial septectomy or catheter septostomy with stenting, to allow these unstable infants to stabilize before definitive therapy. Kumar et al,[9] in a retrospective study, reported that a prenatal diagnosis of this condition improves the preoperative condition of the neonate but may not significantly alter the outcome of management.

EVOLUTION OF STAGED SURGICAL MANAGEMENT

Among the earliest reports of attempted palliation of HLHS were those of Cayler et al[10] in 1970 and Freedom et al[11] in 1977, which both described right and left branch pulmonary artery banding, together with the use of a Waterston shunt in one instance and a Pott's shunt in the other. The durability of these palliations were 7 and 16 months, respectively, in these 2 babies with critical aortic stenosis in the first, and aortic atresia and ventricular septal defect in the second. Separate banding of the branch pulmonary arteries resulted in distortion of the distal pulmonary arteries and maldistribution of flow. Both children died without more definitive surgery. Litwin et al[12] in 1972 performed an operation for interrupted aortic arch in which a nonvalved conduit was placed from the proximal main pulmonary artery to the descending thoracic aorta, and the main pulmonary artery was banded distal to the conduit. The one survivor manifested severe distortion of pulmonary arteries and developed pulmonary vascular obstructive disease. Several surgeons reported the use of similar operations in an effort to treat neonates with HLHS. These included Albert and Bryant[13] in 1978, and Mohri et al[14] in Japan in 1979.

Doty et al[15] in 1977 reported on efforts at surgical repair of HLHS in 5 neonates. A Dacron graft was used to connect the main pulmonary artery to the aorta, and the branch pulmonary arteries were connected to the right atrium using a second Dacron graft. All 5 of the patients died, probably because the high pulmonary vascular resistance of the neonate precluded adequate flow of systemic venous blood from the right atrium to the pulmonary arteries.

Norwood's early efforts at palliative surgery for HLHS included an operation performed in November 1977 that encompassed enlargement of the atrial septal defect, a modified Glenn shunt, ligation of the patent ductus arteriosus, left pulmonary artery banding, and side-to-side anastomosis of the aortic arch with the main pulmonary artery by using the right pulmonary artery to extend the angioplasty. This patient died 7 hours after surgery, probably because of the high pulmonary vascular resistance. The first successful repair of HLHS with long-term survival was reported by Norwood et al[16] in 1980. That procedure included the use of a 10-mm Dacron graft placed from the main pulmonary artery to the descending thoracic aorta. The patent ductus arteriosus was ligated, and a band was placed around the main pulmonary artery distal to the graft. The operation had to be revised 2 weeks later because of distal migration of the band resulting in right pulmonary artery occlusion. During the revision, a conduit was placed from the right ventricular outflow tract to the descending aorta. This resulted in the first reported case of long-term survival after palliation of HLHS (Fig 1). From these early efforts of

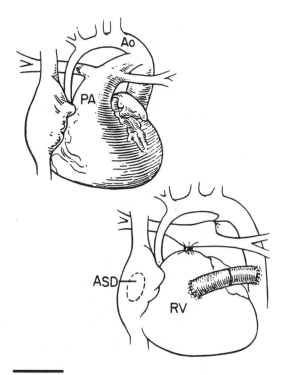

FIGURE 1.

Norwood's original description of his technique in 1980. A conduit was placed between main pulmonary artery *(PA)* and descending thoracic aorta *(Ao)*, and distal main pulmonary artery was banded to limit pulmonary blood flow. Ductus was ligated. *Abbreviations: RV,* Right ventricle; *ASD,* atrial septal defect. (Courtesy of Norwood WI, Kirklin JK, Sanders SP: Hypoplastic left heart syndrome: Experience with palliative surgery. *Am J Cardiol* 45:87-91. Copyright 1980 by Excerpta Medica, Inc. Reprinted by permission.)

Norwood's, it became clear that the essential ingredients of initial palliation of HLHS included establishment of a permanent communication between the right ventricle and the aorta, limitation of pulmonary blood flow to attenuate pulmonary vascular changes caused by elevated pulmonary blood flow and pressure, and insurance of a satisfactory interatrial communication. During the same era, several other surgeons published isolated reports of similar palliative approaches. Doty et al[17] in 1980 described an operation that included the creation of a calibrated opening in the graft connecting the main pulmonary artery to the aorta, with this opening connecting to the pulmonary arteries and thus limiting pulmonary blood flow. Levitsky et al[18] in 1980 described the use of Litwin's operation to repair a case of aortic atresia.

In 1983, Norwood's group[19] reported a further evolution of their approach to palliation, and this included all the features of what has become known as the Norwood stage 1 palliative procedure. Cardiopulmonary bypass was established by cannulation of the main pulmonary artery for arterial infusion, and the right atrial appendage for venous return. The body was cooled to 20°C, and circulatory arrest was established. An anastomosis was performed between the divided proximal main pulmonary artery and the ascending aorta and aortic arch. A 4-mm shunt of polytetrafluoroethylene (PTFE) was placed between the new ascending aorta and the branch pulmonary arteries. Norwood hypothesized that the use of autologous vascular tissue and of the normally developed pulmonary valve in the systemic circulation would maximize both the technical simplicity of the procedure and the potential for growth and development of the reconstructed great vessels (Fig 2). The patient made a rather uneventful recovery and eventually, in 1982, underwent a second reconstructive procedure. The pulmonary and systemic circulations were separated by partitioning the atrium in such a fashion that the pulmonary venous return was directed to the tricuspid valve, and the right atrium was anastomosed directly to the branch pulmonary arteries. The shunt was removed. After this modified Fontan procedure, the patient had minimal pleural effusions in the postoperative period that subsequently resolved. The patient was discharged 21 days after the operation.

As they gained experience with treatment of a large volume of infants with this anomaly, Norwood's group noted some problems from their earlier cases, including development of aortic arch obstruction and pulmonary artery distortion. These problems were addressed by devising some technical modifications to their origi-

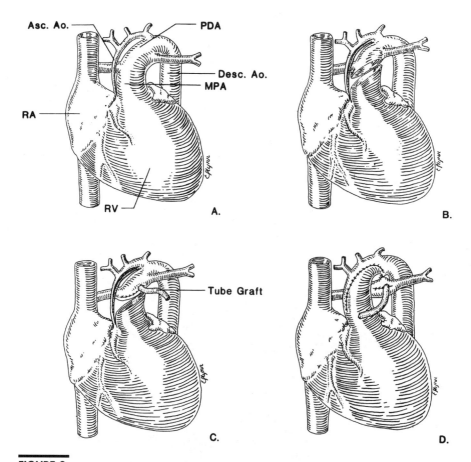

FIGURE 2.

Norwood's modification in 1983 of his original technique. Direct aortopulmonary anastomosis without the use of homograft patch and a central shunt was performed. *Abbreviations: RA,* Right atrium; *Ao,* aorta; *PDA,* patent ductus arteriosus; *MPA,* main pulmonary artery; *RV,* right ventricle. (Reprinted by permission of *The New England Journal of Medicine,* courtesy of Norwood WI, Lang P, Hansen DD: Physiologic repair of aortic atresia–hypoplastic left heart syndrome. *N Engl J Med* 308:23-26. Copyright 1983, Massachusetts Medical Society. All rights reserved.)

nal procedures. A variety of methods were used to construct the shunt, including a modified Blalock-Taussig shunt and a central shunt (Fig 3). Patch material was used to augment the neoaorta from the point of amalgamation of the proximal main pulmonary artery with the aorta, through the length of the aortic arch and down to the descending thoracic aorta beyond the point of insertion of the ductus. Pigott and Norwood et al[20] reported experience with a large volume of patients (104 cases) in 1988. Patients in this series ranged in weight from 1.7 to 4.2 kg, and had a median age of 6 days. Ninety-two of the 104 infants had normally related great arteries with aortic atresia or aortic stenosis and hypoplasia of the left ventricle. Ten had a complete common atrioventricular canal defect with marked malalignment to the right and resultant left heart hypoplasia. Twelve patients had double-outlet right ventricle with aortic and mitral atresia. The ascending aorta was estimated to have a diameter of 1 to 4 mm, with a median diameter of 2 mm. Four patients in this series had associated cardiac anomalies: 3 had total anomalous pulmonary

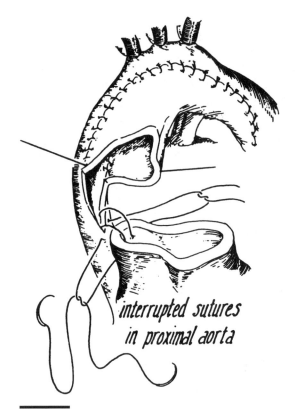

FIGURE 3.

Norwood's modification in 1988 using homograft patch to augment aortic arch and incorporating this onto aortopulmonary anastomosis. This modification was introduced to prevent aortic arch obstruction seen earlier in the series. Central shunt was used in this modification. (Courtesy of Pigott JD, Murphy JD, Barber G, et al: Palliative reconstructive surgery for hypoplastic left heart syndrome. *Ann Thorac Surg* 45:122-128, 1988. Reprinted with permission from the Society of Thoracic Surgeons.)

venous connection of the supracardiac type and 1 had VATER (vertebral, anal, tracheo-esophageal, and renal anomalies) association.

NORWOOD'S FIRST STAGE PALLIATION

Surface cooling is initiated by maintaining the operating room at approximately 55°F (Fig 4). After the induction of general endotracheal anesthesia, a cooling blanket is used and bags of crushed ice are placed around the infant's head. Midline sternotomy and partial thymectomy are performed. With minimal manipulation of the heart, the main pulmonary artery is cannulated just above the sinuses of Valsalva. A single venous cannula is inserted through the right atrial appendage. With the establishment of cardiopulmonary bypass at a flow of 150 to 200 mL/kg per minute, the right and left pulmonary arterial branches are occluded with snares, to ensure optimal systemic perfusion through the ductus arteriosus. During the period of cooling and perfusion, the branch vessels of the aortic arch are exposed and are looped with suture tourniquets in preparation for circulatory arrest. Once cooling to the desired temperature has been accomplished (nasopharyngeal temperature of 18C° to 20°C), the branch vessels of the aortic arch are occluded with the suture tourniquets, and the circulation is discontinued. Blood is drained through the venous cannula into the bypass reservoir, and the cannulas are removed. Atrial septectomy is performed. In most instances, exposure through the right atrial cannulation site is sufficient to visualize and excise septum primum. Occasionally a separate atriotomy is performed, which may be important when the atrial septum is particularly thick or when there is marked leftward deviation of the superior posterior attachment of septum primum. The main pulmonary artery is transected just proximal to the origin of the right branch pulmonary artery. The distal opening in the main pulmonary artery is closed with an oval patch of pulmonary homograft arterial tissue. The ductus arteriosus is exposed by proximal traction on the pulmonary arteries. The ductus is isolated, ligated, and transected at its entrance into the thoracic aorta. The thoracic aorta is incised medially. This incision is carried along the lesser curvature of the aortic arch into the ascending aorta to a level adjacent to the point of transection of the proximal main pulmonary artery. Distally, the incision is extended beyond the point of entrance of the ductus arteriosus for a centimeter or more. Ductal tissue is excised. A gusset of previously cryopreserved pulmonary artery homograft vascular tissue is used for aortic arch augmentation as it is thin, pliable, and hemostatic. This suture line is begun distally in the thoracic aorta and contin-

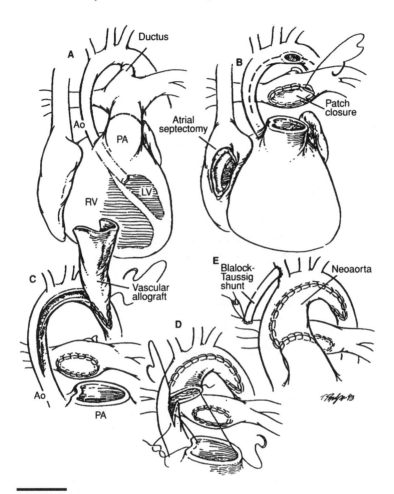

FIGURE 4.
Norwood stage 1 palliation as it is currently performed. Steps in the first stage
palliative procedure, or Norwood operation. **A,** The main pulmonary artery *(PA)*
is transected just proximal to the origins of the branch pulmonary arteries *(dot-
ted line)*. **B,** Atrial septectomy is achieved through the right atrial cannulation
site. The distal main pulmonary artery is closed with an oval patch of cryopreserved pulmonary artery homograft tissue. The ductus arteriosus is transected at
its entrance into the aorta *(Ao)*. An incision is extended both distally and proximally in the aorta. **C,** The aortic arch is augmented with a patch of cryopreserved
pulmonary artery homograft tissue. **D,** Proximally, the aorta is anastomosed to the
adjacent main pulmonary artery with a few interrupted sutures. The homograft
patch is then sutured to the remainder of the circumference of the transected
proximal main pulmonary artery. **E,** A systemic-to-pulmonary artery shunt is constructed usually by interposing a length of 3.5- or 4-mm polytetrafluoroethylene
graft between the innominate artery and the right pulmonary artery. *Abbreviations:
LV,* Left ventricle; *RV,* right ventricle.

ued proximally to augment the aortic arch. The most proximal portion of the gusset is sutured to the transected proximal main pulmonary artery, which has been anastomosed in side-to-side fashion to the ascending aorta. This aortopulmonary anastomosis is a delicate and crucial technical part of the procedure, which in some instances may be best performed by using multiple interrupted sutures. The heart is recannulated and bypass is resumed. The heart generally resumes beating spontaneously, but occasionally requires defibrillation. During the period of perfusion and rewarming, a systemic to pulmonary artery shunt is constructed. Although this is generally accomplished by interposition of a PTFE tube graft between the proximal innominate artery and the proximal right branch pulmonary artery, alternative methods may be applicable (including the use of a central shunt from the underside of the augmented aortic arch to the confluence of the pulmonary arteries). The branch pulmonary arteries or the shunt itself are maintained occluded until the patient has been fully rewarmed. At this point, ventilation is commenced and the shunt is opened to provide pulmonary blood flow. Separation from cardiopulmonary bypass is generally accomplished with minimal inotropic support. Ventilation is accomplished with the FIO_2 gradually being reduced to the lowest level that results in satisfactory oxygenation (systemic arterial saturation, 70%-80%).

INTERMEDIATE PALLIATION

Among the principal goals of the initial palliative procedure are the preservation of ventricular function and of the integrity of the pulmonary vasculature, to prepare the child for eventual separation of the pulmonary and systemic circulations by means of a modification of the Fontan procedure. In the early experience with conversion from the palliated state to the Fontan-type connection, it was observed that even among those infants who were well palliated, there were many who went on to develop a low cardiac output state early after the Fontan procedure. This low output state was often characterized by tachycardia and only transient cardiac output response to volume loading, with the observation that ventricular filling pressures became progressively higher and third spacing of fluid increased. Echocardiographic examination of some of these patients revealed a very high ratio of ventricular wall thickness to cavity volume: that is, a very contracted ventricle that had become very hypertrophied, stiff, and poorly filled. It became evident that this was reflective of a change in ventricular geometry that accompanied the process of reducing the volume work of the single ventricle from that of both the pulmonary and systemic circulations, to that of the systemic circulation alone. This phenomenon was accompanied by a high operative mortality for the Fontan procedure. It was hypothesized that the abrupt reduction of volume work after the Fontan procedure resulted in persistence of an increased muscle mass in the setting of an acutely diminished volume of the ventricular cavity. This led us to believe that dividing the Fontan operation into 2 procedures could accomplish earlier reduction of the volume work of the single ventricle, and would allow normalization of the ventricular mass to volume ratio before completion of the Fontan operation. This then, would minimize the impact of changes in ventricular geometry on outcome and survival.

Intermediate palliation is accomplished using 1 of 2 surgical techniques. Superior cavopulmonary anastomosis (the bidirectional Glenn shunt) is performed by transecting the superior vena cava, creating an end-to-side anastomosis of the superior vena to the right pulmonary artery, closure of the cardiac end of the superior vena cava, interruption of the azygous vein, and elimination of the systemic to pulmonary artery shunt. This usually is accomplished using cardiopulmonary bypass or circulatory arrest. There have been reports of this type of procedure being performed with a temporary shunt from the superior vena cava to the right atrium, avoiding the use of cardiopulmonary bypass.

The hemi-Fontan was introduced in 1989 as the first step in a 2-staged approach to the Fontan operation.[21] The principles of the hemi-Fontan operation include connection of the superior vena cava to the pulmonary arteries, elimination of the systemic to pulmonary shunt, elimination of other sources of antegrade flow to the pulmonary arteries, augmentation of the central pulmonary arteries to eliminate stenosis or distortion, and maintenance of physical continuity between the heart and the superior cavopulmonary amalgamation, facilitating the eventual completion Fontan operation.

TECHNIQUE OF HEMI-FONTAN OPERATION

The hemi-Fontan procedure is performed through a median sternotomy with the use of cardiopulmonary bypass and a brief period of deep hypothermic circulatory arrest (Fig 5).[21] After cardioplegic arrest, an incision is made in the most superior portion of the right atrium and carried superiorly onto the medial aspect of the right superior vena cava. The branch pulmonary arteries are opened anteriorly from a point just medial to the upper lobe

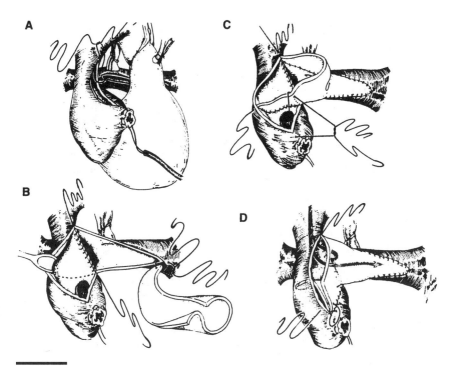

FIGURE 5.
Hemi-Fontan operation. **A,** The systemic-to-pulmonary artery shunt is occluded and may be excised. The confluence of the pulmonary arteries is opened anteriorly. **B,** The right superior vena cava and right pulmonary artery are anastomosed to one another in side-to-side fashion. **C,** A gusset of cryopreserved pulmonary artery homograft tissue is used to augment the confluence of the pulmonary arteries to create a roof over the large anastomosis of the superior vena cava to the pulmonary arteries and as a dam to close the surgically enlarged junction of the right atrium with the right superior vena cava. **D,** Flow from the superior vena cava is into the right and left branch pulmonary arteries, as indicated by the *arrows*. (Courtesy of Jacobs M: Hypoplastic left heart syndrome, in Kaiser LR, Kron IL, Spray TL (eds): *Mastery of Caradiothoracic Surgery.* Philadelphia, Lippincott-Raven, 1998.)

branch on the right side to a corresponding point just proximal to the upper lobe branch on the left side. The right superior vena cava is anastomosed in side-to-side fashion to the right pulmonary artery. If there is a left superior vena cava, this is associated in similar fashion with the left pulmonary artery. A patch of pulmonary artery homograft vascular tissue is used to augment the confluence of the pulmonary arteries anteriorly, to create a roof over the anastomosis of the superior vena cava with the branch pulmonary arteries, and to create a dam, occluding the inflow of the superior vena cava into the right atrium. This effectively enlarges the junction of the superior vena cava with the right atrium to a caliber equivalent to that of the junction of the inferior vena cava with the right atrium, but temporarily occludes this connection until it is reopened at the time of the completion Fontan procedure.

Additional procedures may be accomplished at the time of the hemi-Fontan operation, to facilitate optimal outcome from the eventual completion Fontan procedure. In a series of 400 hemi-Fontan operations reported by Jacobs et al,[21] associated procedures included atrial septectomy (17 patients), relief of aortic arch obstruction (13 patients), repair of anomalous pulmonary venous connections (6 patients), and atrioventricular valvuloplasty (6 patients), and others. Interposition of the hemi-Fontan operation between the Norwood stage 1 palliation and the Fontan operation has resulted in a larger percentage of patients ultimately coming to complete physiologic repair via the Fontan operation. It has been observed that although the volume work of the ventricle is reduced from pumping both pulmonary and systemic blood flow to systemic blood flow only at the time of the hemi-Fontan operation (just as it is with a one-stage Fontan operation), the low-output state associated with a contracted ventricular cavity volume is only rarely observed and considerably less lethal after the hemi-Fontan operation than it is after a primary Fontan operation. This is partly because only superior vena caval flow must traverse the pulmonary vascular bed, with inferior vena caval return going directly to the systemic ventricle. Thus, there is less impediment to ventricular filling, and cardiac output is preserved. Also, serial echocardiographic examination of patients undergoing staged reconstruction has shown that the degree of change in the ratio of wall thickness to cavity size is of lesser magnitude after the hemi-Fontan operation than it is after a primary Fontan procedure.[21] The other potential advantages of a 2-stage approach to the Fontan procedure include elimination of traditional Fontan risk factors such as pulmonary artery distortion, pulmonary artery stenosis, atrioventricular valve regurgitation, and elimination of other sources of pulmonary blood flow. Introduction of the hemi-Fontan procedure in preparation for the completion Fontan resulted in a decrease in operative mortality for the Fontan procedure from 16% to 8%.[22]

THE COMPLETION FONTAN OPERATION

Management of patients after stage 1 palliation involves eventual creation of a Fontan circulation with the goals of reduction to normal of the volume work of the single ventricle, and achievement of normal or near-normal systemic arterial saturation. As previously mentioned, the hemi-Fontan operation is designed in a such a way that the subsequent completion Fontan is a straightforward technical exercise.

TECHNIQUE OF THE COMPLETION FONTAN PROCEDURE

The completion Fontan procedure is usually performed 12 to 18 months after the hemi-Fontan operation (Fig 6). After median sternotomy, minimal dissection is needed to make preparations for cardiopulmonary bypass. The aorta and right atrium are cannulated, and hypothermic bypass is established. During cooling, enough of the aorta is mobilized to afford access for aortic cross-clamping. The free wall of the right atrium is carefully dissected from the adjacent

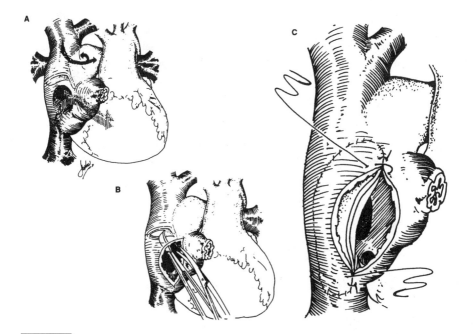

FIGURE 6.

Completion Fontan procedure. **A,** Before the completion Fontan procedure, only superior vena caval flow enters the branch pulmonary arteries. Inferior vena caval flow and pulmonary venous return enter the systemic ventricle. **B,** The homograft dam, which was previously placed to occlude the junction of the right atrium with the right superior vena cava, is widely excised. **C,** Total caval pulmonary connection is accomplished by a lateral atrial tunnel technique. The lateral atrial tunnel is composed medially of a gusset of polytetrafluoroethylene and laterally of native atrial wall. (Courtesy of Jacobs ML: Hypoplastic left heart syndrome, in Kaiser LR, Kron IL, Spray TL (eds): *Mastery of Caradiothoracic Surgery.* Philadelphia, Lippincott-Raven, 1998.)

pericardium. Cooling is continued until the nasopharyngeal temperature has reached 18°C. When the desired temperature is reached, the aorta is cross-clamped and cardioplegic solution is infused. Cannulas are retrieved. An incision is made in the free wall of the right atrium, parallel and slightly anterior to the sulcus terminalis. The incision extends inferiorly to the level of the eustachian valve of the inferior vena cava, and superiorly to within a few millimeters of the junction of the right atrium with the superior vena cava. The dam of homograft tissue that was previously placed to separate the right atrium from the confluence of the superior vena cava and pulmonary arteries is excised. Lateral tunnel cavopulmonary connection is performed by using a gusset of PTFE. In our practice, this is generally trimmed from a 10-mm graft that has been split longitudinally. The gusset is sewn inferiorly around the opening of the inferior vena cava into the right atrium, and then along the interior atrial wall just anterior to the edge of the atrial septal defect. Superiorly, the gusset is sewn to the edges of the opening into the superior vena cava and pulmonary arteries. The lateral tunnel is then completed by incorporating the anterior edge of the PTFE gusset in the closure of the atriotomy incision. In most instances we choose to fenestrate the lateral tunnel. There is now considerable evidence that the right-to-left shunt accomplished by fenestration results in better preservation of ventricular filling, and thus improves cardiac output in the early postoperative period. It also appears that this strategy is associated with less morbidity from effusions. Because a single large fenestration may remain patent for a considerable time and require device closure, we have chosen to use multiple small fenestrations. Early in our experience, these were created by puncturing the PTFE graft with a 14-gauge needle. This did not prove to be entirely reliable, and thus in the last 100 cases we have created 3 separate fenestrations with a 2.5-mm aortic punch. These multiple small fenestrations gradually close, thus affording the advantages of a right-to-left shunt in the early postoperative period, without the persistence of a significant right-to-left shunt at late follow-up. In virtually all cases, the arterial saturation in room air is above 90% at 6 months after the completion Fontan procedure.[23]

Early in our experience, the lateral tunnel completion Fontan was modified with the goal of accomplishing partial exclusion of hepatic veins from the systemic venous pathway. This technique, which was independently introduced by both Norwood and LeCompte, resulted early postoperatively in a right-to-left shunt of magnitude similar to that accomplished by fenestration. The incidence of persistent pleural effusions was extremely low in patients who underwent Fontan procedures with partial hepatic vein exclusion. However, a significant number of the patients developed increasing cyanosis months to years after surgery, as a result of increasing diversion of systemic venous blood flow from the lateral tunnel via the excluded hepatic veins. Many of these patients required either operative revision or a catheterization laboratory intervention to occlude intrahepatic veno-venous connections.

More recent modifications to the completion Fontan procedure for patients with HLHS include the extracardiac Fontan procedure, accomplished with or without cardiopulmonary bypass. The extracardiac Fontan procedure involves the interposition of a prosthetic conduit or aortic homograft conduit between the divided inferior vena cava and the pulmonary arteries. This can be performed either with or without fenestration. Fenestration is accomplished either by excising adjacent buttons from the medial aspect of the conduit and from the atrial free wall and creating a "window," or by interposing a small PTFE tube graft between the large conduit and the right atrium. When the second stage procedure has been a hemi-Fontan procedure, fenestration can be accomplished in the setting of an extracardiac conduit Fontan by creating a calibrated opening in the homograft dam separating the superior vena cava and pulmonary arteries from the right atrium.[24] The extracardiac completion Fontan procedure can also be accomplished without the use of cardiopulmonary bypass in selected cases.[24] A tube graft is anastomosed end-to-side to the right pulmonary artery after selectively directing flow from the superior vena cava to the left pulmonary artery with an appropriately curved vascular clamp. Subsequently, an inferior vena cava to right atrial shunt is placed. The inferior vena cava is divided. The cardiac end is oversewn. The inferior vena cava is then anastomosed to the lower end of the conduit, creating an extracardiac total cavopulmonary connection. Proponents of this modification observe "better early postoperative hemodynamics" after total cavopulmonary connection without bypass, as compared with their own patients undergoing a conventional Fontan procedure with cardiopulmonary bypass.

RECENT DEVELOPMENTS IN STAGED SURGICAL RECONSTRUCTION

Although Norwood's stage 1 palliation has been adopted by most proponents of reconstructive surgical therapy for HLHS, several technical modifications have been introduced. Some are intended primarily to minimize the adverse effects of cardiopulmonary bypass, hypothermic circulatory arrest, or both. Some are intended to simplify the technical performance of the initial palliative procedure.

NEW BYPASS TECHNIQUES

As increasing experience has led to improved rates of survival from staged reconstructive surgery for HLHS, increasing emphasis is placed on neurologic outcome, and the potential for injury associated with bypass, deep hypothermia, and circulatory arrest. Evidence of overt brain injury may be found in up to 10% of children, with subtle neuropsychiatric injury reported in up to 50%.[25-27] The pathology of brain injury includes cerebral necrosis, periventricular leukomalacia, brain stem necrosis, and intracranial hemorrhage. Numerous surgical teams have revised the technical aspects of the palliative operation to minimize the duration of hypothermic circulatory arrest.[28]

Selective Cerebral Perfusion

Asou et al[29] in 1996 described a technique of selective cerebral perfusion applicable to the initial palliative operation for HLHS (Fig 7). Cardiopulmonary bypass is established as usual by pulmonary artery and atrial cannulation. During the period of cooling, a 4-mm PTFE graft is anastomosed to the innominate artery, and this is connected to the arterial cannula by a Y-connector. After systemic cooling has been accomplished, the arterial cannula to the main pulmonary artery is clamped and removed, and the innominate artery is occluded proximal to the site of shunt insertion. Perfusion via the innominate artery is maintained at 50 mL/kg per minute, and arterial pressure is monitored in the left temporal artery. After completion of the arch reconstruction, flow is increased to a level of 150 mL/kg per minute for whole-body perfusion. The neoaorta is recannulated, and the cannula into the PTFE graft is occluded and removed. Finally, the PTFE graft is trimmed and anastomosed to the pulmonary artery to complete the systemic to pulmonary artery shunt. A variation of this technique involving direct aortic cannulation has been used in patients whose ascending aorta is at the large end of the spectrum of HLHS. Asou[29] used these techniques in 8 neonates with HLHS, and 5 survived. Pigula et al[30] applied similar methods of selective cerebral perfusion and measured cerebral blood volume and oxygen saturation with near infrared spectroscopy. A brief period of total circulatory arrest was used during the period of exchange of arterial perfusion cannulas between the pulmonary artery and the PTFE graft to the innominate artery. Pigula found that regional cerebral flow at a level of 20 mL/kg per minute, with clamping of the descending thoracic aorta, resulted in a cerebral blood volume index and an oxygen saturation that were comparable with those

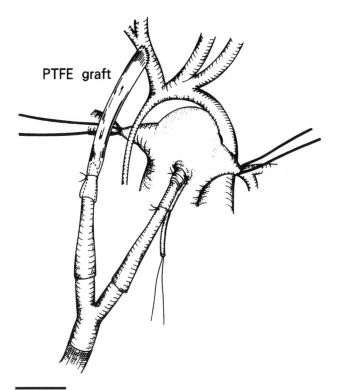

PTFE graft

FIGURE 7.
Asou et al from Japan in 1996 described selective cerebral perfusion via a polytetrafluoroethylene *(PTFE)* graft anastomosed to the innominate artery, during the period of circulatory arrest. A Y-connector was placed in the arterial line for this purpose. (Courtesy of Asou T, Kado H, Imoto Y, et al: Selective cerebral perfusion technique during aortic arch repair in neonates. *Ann Thorac Surg* 61:1546-1548, 1996. Reprinted with permission from the Society of Thoracic Surgeons.)

observed during whole-body perfusion before the institution of regional perfusion and circulatory arrest (Fig 8). This corroborates earlier experimental work by Swain et al[31] in sheep which showed that 10 mL/kg per minute of cerebral blood flow was sufficient to preserve cerebral high-energy substrates. A variety of technical modifications have been used by other surgeons to accomplish regional cerebral perfusion in neonates. McElhinney et al[32] cannulated the proximal innominate artery directly. Thus, they avoided the brief period of hypothermic circulatory arrest required to transfer the cannula from the PTFE graft to the main pulmonary artery. Tchervenkov suggested cannulating the aorta at the base of the innominate artery

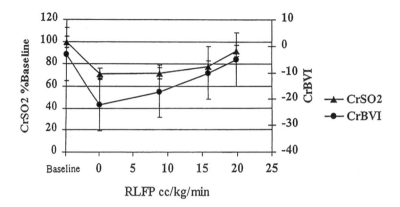

FIGURE 8.
Relative cerebral volume index *(CrBVI)* and oxygen saturation *(CrSO$_2$)* as a function of regional low-flow perfusion rate. Reacquisition of baseline CrBVI occurs consistently at about 20 mL . kg^{-1} . min^{-1}, and is mirrored by return to baseline CrSO$_2$. (Courtesy of Pigula FA, Nemoto EM, Griffith BP, et al: Regional low-flow perfusion provides cerebral circulatory support during neonatal aortic arch reconstruction. *J Thorac Cardiovasc Surg* 119:333, 2000.)

and advancing the cannula tip into the proximal innominate artery for regional cerebral perfusion only during the period of arch reconstruction (personal communication). Obviously, there are concerns that direct cannulation of the tiny innominate or carotid arteries may ultimately result in some stenosis of these vessels.

First Stage Palliation Without Circulatory Arrest
Recently, 2 different techniques have been described to perform first stage palliative procedures without using circulatory arrest. Kishimoto et al[33] reported a technique of performing a stage 1 palliation on a beating heart. Median sternotomy was performed, and the innominate artery was cannulated with a 2.1-mm metal cannula. Another cannula was placed in the descending thoracic aorta. After dissection, a crossclamp was placed on the proximal aortic arch to maintain coronary and cerebral perfusion via the innominate artery cannula. The left carotid and subclavian arteries were occluded. The pulmonary trunk was divided proximal to the origin of the right pulmonary artery, and was connected to the aortic arch by using a xenopericardial graft without enlargement of the ascending aorta. A 6-mm xenopericardial conduit with a bicuspid valve was interposed between the right ventricle via ventriculotomy and the pulmonary arteries, to provide pulmonary blood

flow. Seven patients underwent this procedure between 1992 and 1999. Although there were no early mortalities in this group, 1 patient died at 2 months of conduit stenosis and hypoxia, and 2 more patients died of heart failure 4 and 29 months after the operation. Only 1 patient in the series underwent a second stage reconstructive procedure (Glenn) 5 months after the initial operation. A major drawback of this technique is the use of a ventriculotomy in the systemic ventricle of a single ventricle circulation.

Imoto et al[34] in 1999 also reported efforts to achieve initial palliation without circulatory arrest. A PTFE graft was anastomosed to the innominate artery and used as the site of arterial inflow for cardiopulmonary bypass, with bicaval cannulation (Fig 9). Elevation of the heart from the pericardial space allowed access to the descending thoracic aorta in the posterior mediastinum for place-

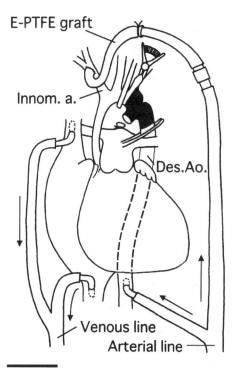

FIGURE 9.

Lower body perfusion by cannulation of descending thoracic aorta *(Des Ao)* in the pericardial sac combined with cerebral perfusion. *Abbreviation: E-PTFE,* Expanded polytetrafluoroethylene. (Courtesy of Imoto Y, Kado H, Yasui H, et al: Norwood procedure without circulatory arrest. *J Thorac Cardiovasc Surg* 68:559-561, 1999.)

ment of a second arterial inflow cannula. Pump flows of 180 mL/kg per minute were used with cooling to 30.4°C. After clamping the distal arch, the left subclavian artery, and descending thoracic aorta, the ductus arteriosus was ligated and anastomosis was performed between the thoracic aorta and the arch. The undersurface of the aortic arch was incised, and the incision extended onto the ascending aorta. Under cardioplegic arrest, the neoaorta was constructed with direct anastomosis of the proximal pulmonary trunk to the ascending aorta and aorta arch. The PTFE graft was subsequently disconnected from the arterial inflow cannula, trimmed, and anastomosed to the pulmonary artery. The case report indicated that the patient was well 5 months after this initial palliative procedure.

MODIFIED NORWOOD PROCEDURE WITHOUT AORTIC PATCH AUGMENTATION

While Norwood and his associates have for more than a decade continued to use pulmonary artery homograft vascular tissue to augment the aortic reconstruction, others have returned to Norwood's earlier technique of pulmonary artery to aortic amalgamation and arch reconstruction using only autologous tissue. Fraser and Mee[28] in 1995 reported the use of such a procedure in 13 neonates (Fig 10). Arterial inflow was accomplished by direct cannulation of the ductus arteriosus in most patients, and of the ascending aorta in those with a larger aorta. After the initiation of cardiopulmonary bypass, the ductus was divided proximally, eliminating pulmonary blood flow and ensuring satisfactory systemic perfusion. The main pulmonary artery was transected obliquely beginning just proximal to the right pulmonary orifice. An autologous pericardial patch was used to close the opening in the pulmonary artery bifurcation. A PTFE shunt was interposed between the innominate artery and the right branch pulmonary artery. The proximal descending thoracic aortic and arch vessels were extensively mobilized. After excision of all ductal tissue, the thoracic aorta was anastomosed to the undersurface of the aortic arch. The proximal main pulmonary artery was incorporated into the anastomosis between the arch and the descending thoracic aorta. The mean circulatory arrest time in this group of patients was 32 minutes. Seven patients underwent cardiac catheterization at 2 to 4 months postoperatively and showed no evidence of recurrent aortic coarctation or left pulmonary artery stenosis. There was evidence of coronary ischemia in 2 patients who required revision, and suspicion of coronary ischemia in 1 patient who died. In these patients,

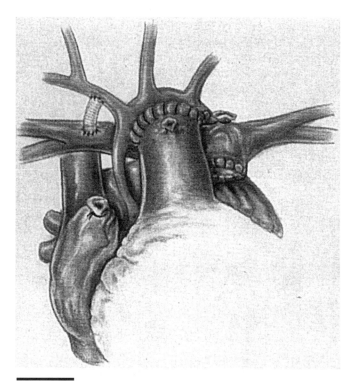

FIGURE 10.
Modified Norwood procedure with autologous great vessel tissue only. A 3.0 to 4.0 mm water repellant fabric (Gore-Tex) shunt provides pulmonary blood flow. (Courtesy of Fraser CD Jr, Mee RBB: Modified Norwood procedure for hypoplastic left heart syndrome. *Ann Thorac Surg* 60:546S-549S, 1995. Reprinted with permission from the Society of Thoracic Surgeons.)

there was probably some limitation of flow into the long ascending aorta, which was not incised and enlarged as in Norwood's stage 1 palliation. In the 2 patients who were successfully revised, the ascending aorta was divided and translocated to the innominate artery, with resolution of coronary ischemia. Proponents of this technique emphasized the advantage of the shortened circulatory arrest time. The role of this technique in terms of its long-term effects on aortic arch growth and coronary perfusion requires further evaluation. A variety of minor technical modifications have been proposed to address the issue of kinking or stenosis, limiting inflow into the tiny ascending aorta and thus resulting in myocardial ischemia.

Ishino et al[35] from Birmingham, England reported a large experience using a technique similar to that described above (Fig 11).

In 120 cases they achieved early survival in 68%. In most patients, all ductal tissue was excised, and the descending aorta was anastomosed to the aortic arch and proximal main pulmonary artery as above. In 22 patients, continuity of the aortic arch was maintained, and the proximal main pulmonary artery was anastomosed directly to the opening in the arch. The incidence of neo–aortic arch obstruction was 23%. At the time of the report, 71 patients in this group had undergone a second stage bidirectional Glenn procedure, and 3 patients had undergone a completion Fontan procedure. In this report, circulatory arrest times varied from 57 to 105 minutes. There was significant interval mortality between the stage 1 palliation and second stage reconstruction, which raised suspicion concerning the adequacy of coronary perfusion in patients

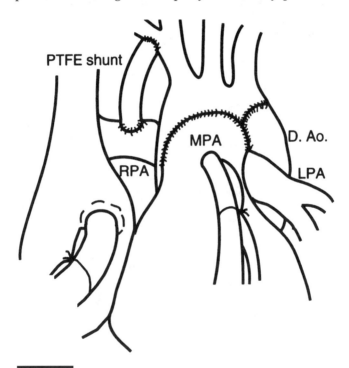

FIGURE 11.
Modified Norwood procedure with autologous tissue. *Abbreviations: PTFE,* polytetrafluoroethylene; *RPA,* right pulmonary artery; *MPA,* main pulmonary artery; *D. Ao.,* descending aorta; *LPA,* left pulmonary artery. (Courtesy of Ishino K, Stumper O, Brawn WJ, et al: The modified Norwood procedure for hypoplastic left heart syndrome: Early to intermediate results of 120 patients with particular reference to aortic arch repair. *J Thorac Cardiovasc Surg* 117:920-930, 1999.)

whose diminutive ascending aorta had not been augmented. It is curious that these procedures which use only autologous tissue are frequently referred to as "modified Norwood operations," because the initial stage 1 palliation described by Norwood[19] in 1983 was accomplished in just this fashion.

Another technical modification, which has not achieved wide acceptance, was described by Pridjian et al[36] in 1995. Anastomosis of the dome of the pulmonary artery to the undersurface of the transverse arch was performed, with placement of a fenestrated patch within the main pulmonary artery to divide systemic and pulmonary blood flow. Two patients underwent this procedure with early survival.

RECENT ADVANCES IN PERIOPERATIVE MANAGEMENT

The recognition of the dynamic nature of the balance between systemic and pulmonary blood flow after initial palliation has given rise to numerous strategies to stabilize this balance and to optimize systemic perfusion. Schmidt et al[37] described the use of an adjustable tourniquet around the modified Blalock-Taussig shunt to limit pulmonary blood flow in the immediate postoperative period. They were able to adjust the degree to which the tourniquet narrowed the shunt when necessary (2 of 7 patients) and achieve consistent survival in a small group of patients by using this technique.

Norwood's group[38] in 1991 described the first clinical use of carbon dioxide added to the inspired gases, to manipulate postoperative hemodynamics in patients undergoing stage 1 Norwood procedures. The role of carbon dioxide as a potent pulmonary vasoconstrictor had earlier been demonstrated by Morray et al.[39] The physiology of patients with HLHS both before and after stage 1 palliation depends on maintenance of a satisfactory balance between systemic and pulmonary resistance. Gullquist et al[40] in 1992 compared 50 neonates undergoing stage 1 palliation with postoperative use of carbon dioxide, with 50 patients managed without this intervention. Early postoperative mortality was significantly less in the patients in the carbon dioxide–treated group. Although alternative strategies have also been used successfully, we have found the use of carbon dioxide in the inspired gases to be a predictable and manageable form of therapy to limit excessive pulmonary blood flow before, during, and after palliative surgery for HLHS. Early attempts at controlling pulmonary overcirculation and achieving hypercarbia by decreasing minute ventilation, resulted in decreased functional residual capacity, with the closure of small airways, atelectasis, and alveolar hypoxemia. Maintaining adequate functional residual capacity with appropriate tidal volumes together with the addition of inspired carbon dioxide minimizes these problems.

A small percentage of patients will have evidence of inadequate pulmonary blood flow after initial palliation. Differential diagnosis in this situation includes inadequacy of the systemic to pulmonary artery shunt (too small or technically unsatisfactory), pulmonary venous obstruction (inadequate atrial septectomy), elevated pulmonary vascular resistance, and inadequate systemic pressure. After ensuring that the shunt is technically adequate, efforts to improve pulmonary blood flow include augmentation of intravascular volume, addition of inotropic support to ensure adequate systemic pressure, lowering the P_{CO_2} by increasing minute ventilation, and increasing the F_{IO_2}. A number of experimental models have been used to recreate and study the physiology of the neonate with a single ventricle and systemic to pulmonary artery shunt. Mora et al[41] created single-ventricle physiology in 18 Yorkshire piglets. The atrial septum was excised. The right ventricle was excluded from the circulation by patch closure of the tricuspid valve, and a 4-mm systemic to pulmonary artery shunt was created. The effect of inspired carbon dioxide on pulmonary vascular resistance and pH was studied. Carbon dioxide was added to the inspired gases in increments of 7 mm Hg up to a level of 35 mm Hg. The pulmonary vascular resistance increased in all animals, in direct correlation with the partial pressure of inspired carbon dioxide (P_{ICO_2}), and inversely with respect to pH (Fig 12). The investigators concluded that the carbon dioxide exerts a vasoactive influence on the pulmonary vasculature that is largely independent of the systemic vascular resistance. Reddy et al[42] created a fetal sheep model of single-ventricle physiology and then postnatally studied the effects of oxygen, nitric oxide, carbon dioxide, and hypoxia on hemodynamics. Nitric oxide and oxygen caused a decrease in pulmonary vascular resistance. Carbon dioxide and hypoxia caused a significant increase in pulmonary vascular resistance, with corresponding changes in the pulmonary/systemic blood flow ratio.

SYSTEMIC OXYGEN DELIVERY

Computer-simulated mathematical models were designed to assess systemic oxygen delivery (D_{O_2}) as a function of arterial oxygen saturation (S_{aO_2}), venous oxygen saturation (S_{vO_2}), systemic arterial-mixed venous oxygen saturation (Sa-v_{O_2}), and (QP/QS).[43] Barnea et al[43] observed that a linear relationship exists between oxygen excess

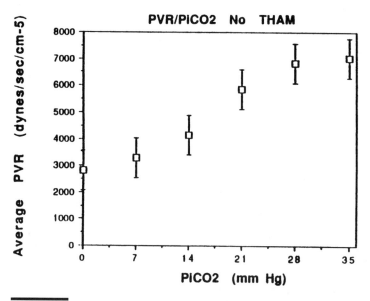

PVR/PICO2 No THAM

FIGURE 12.
Plot of pulmonary vascular resistance *(PVR)* after increments in the partial pressure of inspired carbon dioxide ($PICO_2$), 7 mm Hg each in the group of animals receiving no trishydroxymethylaminomethane *(THAM)*. It shows a direct correlation of PVR with $PICO_2$. (Courtesy of Mora GA, Pizarro C, Jacobs ML, et al: Experimental model of single ventricle: Influence of carbon dioxide on pulmonary vascular dynamics. *Circulation* 90:II-43-II-46, 1994.)

factor (SaO_2/$Sa-vO_2$, mu) and DO_2, and this linear relationship is not altered by changes in cardiac output and pulmonary venous saturation ($SpvO_2$). Interventions that increase oxygen excess factor can be used in clinical situations to optimize systemic oxygen delivery. They advocated the use of continuous monitoring of systemic venous saturation with miniature oximetric catheters. They emphasized that a persistent decrease in SvO_2, even with normal SaO_2 and blood gases, may be an early indicator of excessive pulmonary blood flow.

Others have advocated the use of phenoxybenzamine, an α-adrenergic blocker, as a systemic vasodilator to optimize systemic oxygen delivery in patients undergoing first stage palliation for HLHS. Tweddell et al[44] placed a 4F fiberoptic catheter in the superior vena cava at the time of surgery, and used it postbypass and postoperatively for continuous SvO_2 monitoring. When compared with controls, the group of patients treated with phenoxybenzamine had a higher systemic venous oxygen saturation, narrower arterial venous oxygen content difference, lower ratio of pulmonary to systemic blood flow, and lower indexed systemic vascular resistance. Thus, rather than manipulating the ratio of pulmonary to systemic resistance by increasing pulmonary vascular resistance, these authors chose to balance the circulation and optimize systemic oxygen delivery by lowering the systemic vascular resistance.

Day et al[45] in 1998 reported the use of supplemental nitrogen in newborns with functional single ventricle and ductal-dependent systemic perfusion to prevent pulmonary vascular dilatation. Whereas most of these patients were being managed in anticipation of eventual transplantation, use of nitrogen in the inspired gases without exceeding an FIO_2 of 0.21 helped to prevent excessive pulmonary blood flow in this setting. There was evidence of significant pulmonary vascular disease having developed in one patient. This was not demonstrable in the long-term in the rest of the surviving patients.

BIVENTRICULAR REPAIR

Although the term HLHS generally infers an extreme level of underdevelopment of the left ventricle in the setting of aortic atresia or stenosis, mitral atresia or stenosis, or both, there is certainly a continuous spectrum of left heart underdevelopment (or multiple left heart obstructive lesions) that spans the intermediate ground between HLHS and a fully developed left heart. Kirklin and Barratt-Boyes[46] suggested a classification of HLHS based on the number of obstructive lesions in the left heart complex. Their classification includes 4 levels of left heart obstruction. The first 2 classes include patients with 1 or 2 left-sided obstructive lesions, generally with a normally developed left ventricle. Those in class 3 have 2 or more left-sided obstructive lesions with left ventricular hypoplasia or aortic arch obstruction. Certainly in this group, there are some patients who are best managed by palliation in the style of a Norwood stage 1 procedure. Some, on the other hand, may be able to undergo biventricular repair.

Tchervenkov et al[47] applied the term "hypoplastic left heart complex" for patients in such an intermediate category. In particular, they used this term to describe patients who have no intrinsic aortic valve or mitral valve stenosis, but may have hypoplasia of these structures. This may be associated with varying degrees of ascending aortic and aortic arch hypoplasia, and of small left ventricular size. For patients in this category, Tchervenkov undertook biventricular repair, which included homograft patch enlargement of the ascending aorta and the entire aortic arch and proximal descending thoracic aorta. He described 11 patients treated in this fashion. There were 9 operative survivors and 4 patients who subsequently underwent a total of 6 reoperations for left ventricular outflow tract obstruction. Two patients required prosthetic valve replacement, and 2 patients had 3 operations for recurrent obstruction. Actuarial survival at 8 years was 63%, and freedom from reoperation at 3 years was 25%.

Several sets of criteria have evolved with the intent of predicting likelihood of success with a biventricular repair. Rhodes et al[48] proposed criteria for predicting survival from biventricular repair in patients with critical aortic stenosis. This formulation is based on determinations of indexed mitral valve area, left ventricular long-axis length related to the total length of the heart, and indexed aortic size. Keane et al[49] proposed left ventricular volume assessment and suggested that biventricular repair is less likely to be successful when left ventricular volume is less than 20 mL/m^2 body surface area. Karl et al[50] proposed that when the apex of the heart is not formed by the left ventricle, or the left ventricular size is less than 60% mean for body weight, biventricular repair is less likely to be successful.

Several surgical groups[51] have advocated the use of a Ross-Konno operation for patients with significant left ventricular outflow tract obstruction, borderline left ventricular size, and endocardial fibroelastosis. Presently, there are insufficient data to determine the validity of this approach. Serraf et al[52] reported experience with 21 neonates with ductus-dependent systemic circulation and hypoplastic, but morphologically normal left ventricles. These patients had a mean end-diastolic left ventricular volume of 13.3 ± 3.5 mL/m^2 and a mean Rhodes score of −1.43 ± 0.9. The patients underwent relief of left ventricular outflow obstruction, coarctation repair, closure of atrial septal defect, aortic commissurotomy, and ascending aortic enlargement. There were 3 early and 3 late deaths in this group. The long-term outcome with respect to potential need for reoperations for left ventricular outflow tract obstruction has yet to be determined. Tani et al[53] performed biventricular repair on 20 neonates with duct-dependent systemic circulation and small, but nonstenotic aortic valves. Coarctation repair with arch augmentation was done, and 3 patients underwent pulmonary artery banding with subsequent ventricular septal defect closure. There were no early or late deaths in this series. Subsequent interventions included balloon angioplasty for recurrent aortic obstruction in 2 patients, and resection of subaortic stenosis in 1 patient. The authors conclude that the applicability of Rhodes criteria is limited to those patients with valvar aortic stenosis, and that the criteria do not accurately predict success from biventricular repair in patients with aortic valve hypoplasia (without stenosis) and arch obstruction.

LEFT VENTRICULAR GROWTH

Postnatal growth potential of non–apex-forming left ventricles was evaluated in 6 neonates who were placed on prostaglandin infusions to maintain ductal patency.[54] After 1 month, there were measurable increases in aortic annulus diameter, aortic root diameter, ratio of long axis of the left ventricle to the long axis of the heart, left ventricular end-diastolic volume indexed to body surface area, mitral valve area indexed to body surface area, and Rhodes score. Tricuspid valve area and long axis of the heart indexed to body surface area did not change. Five of the 6 patients underwent biventricular repair, with 1 death. In a similar experience at another center, Foker (personal communication) described experience with 4 neonates with a hypoplastic, but structurally normal left heart. They were managed with partial closure of the interatrial communication, banding of the pulmonary artery, and infusion of prostaglandin to maintain ductal patency. Left ventricular echocardiographic dimensions changed during a 2-week period from 6 SDs below normal to 1 SD below normal. Biventricular repair was undertaken successfully in 2 patients.

RESULTS OF SURGICAL THERAPY
MULTI-INSTITUTION STUDY

In 1998, the Congenital Heart Surgeons Society presented the results of a multi-institutional study of outcomes in managing neonates with aortic atresia. There were 21 participating institutions. A total of 323 neonates with aortic atresia were entered between January 1994 and January 1997. This study examined the prevalence and outcomes of the various treatment strategies. These strategies included staged reconstructive surgery with initial palliation by the Norwood procedure, heart transplantation, and nonsurgical treatment. In this group, 253 patients underwent staged reconstructive surgery, 49 patients underwent heart transplantation, and 21 were in the nonsurgical group. For all patients initially entered into the 2 surgical protocols, survival at 1, 2, and 3 years was 52%, 51%, and 50%, respectively. A multivariate analysis identified incremental risk factors for death at any time after entry to be low birth weight ($P = .04$), associated noncardiac anomaly ($P = .007$), and entry into the nonsurgical protocol ($P < .0001$).

Of the 21 institutions participating in the study, 4 had significantly higher survival statistics. Two of them used the heart transplantation protocol, and 2 institutions used the staged reconstructive surgery protocol. Of the 113 patients treated at these 4 institutions, survival at 1, 2, 3, 12, 24, and 36 months after entry was 77%, 70%, 64%, 62%, and 61%, respectively. It was concluded that aortic size, degree of left ventricular hypoplasia, and degree of mitral hypoplasia or atresia were not predictive of survival from the 2 surgical protocols. The highest survival was achieved with either treatment protocol in an institution strongly committed to the use of one or the other surgical management protocol. Of the 253 patients entered into the staged reconstructive surgery protocol, 140 of them were from 3 large-volume institutions. Two of these institutions were identified as negative risk factors for death at any time after entry. Of the 253 patients entered into the staged reconstructive surgery protocol, 121 patients had subsequently undergone second stage procedures (hemi-Fontan or bidirectional Glenn) at a median age of 6.4 months. Thirty-eight patients had undergone completion Fontan procedure at a median age of 20 months, at the time of the report.

Numerous centers have published individual institutional results of surgical therapy for HLHS. Apart from the previously mentioned results published by Norwood and associates, 2 of the largest institutional series are from the University of Michigan and the Children's Hospital, Boston. Reyes et al[55] described their experience with 253 patients who underwent a Norwood operation for classic HLHS between 1990 and 1997. Hospital survival was 76%. Risk factors for adverse outcome were identified as associated noncardiac congenital conditions ($P = .008$) and severe preoperative obstruction to pulmonary venous return ($P = .03$). Survival after the stage 2 hemi-Fontan operation was 97%. Ninety-four patients underwent a completion Fontan procedure with 88% survival. Survival after the completion Fontan procedure improved significantly when the treatment protocol evolved to include the hemi-Fontan (rather than bidirectional Glenn) as the intermediate procedure. The period of most rapid decline in survival was identified as the first months of life. Most survivors in this series are described as having a normal neurodevelopmental outcome. Forbess et al[56] reported on 212 consecutive patients with HLHS who underwent stage 1 palliative surgery at the Children's Hospital, Boston between 1983 and 1993. The operative mortality in this series was 46.2%. A multivariate analysis revealed better stage 1 operative survival in patients with aortic stenosis and mitral stenosis (P = .006), as opposed to aortic atresia, mitral atresia, or both. Other risk factors identified for stage 1 mortality included lower immediate preoperative pH (P = .03) and weight less than 3 kg (P = .015). Overall first-year survival for patients with mitral stenosis and aortic stenosis was 59%, compared with 33% for all others (P = .001). Risk factors for intermediate death included smaller ascending aorta (P < .001), aortic atresia (P < .001), and mitral atresia (P = .002). In a subsequent report from the same center comparing results of Norwood stage 1 palliation for HLHS to those with lesions other than HLHS, the authors described improved operative survival in the most recent series. There was, however, a significant survival advantage in patients with lesions other than HLHS.[57]

AUTOPSY STUDY

Bartrum et al[58] studied 122 heart specimens of patients who had died after a Norwood stage 1 palliative procedure at the Children's Hospital, Boston, between 1980 and 1995. They concluded that in more than one third of the patients, the cause of death was impairment of coronary perfusion. Precoronary stenosis was present in 26 of the hearts. The opening into the ascending aorta that carries blood flow to the coronary arteries was found to be narrowed. Many of these patients had undergone an operative procedure that did not include a longitudinal incision of the medial aspect of the ascending aorta and amalgamation of the ascending aorta with the proximal pulmonary artery and arch reconstruction. Less common findings included thromboembolism of the right coronary artery, surgical ligation of an aberrant circumflex artery originating from the right coronary artery, extrinsic compression of an intramural right coronary artery by prosthetic material used to augment the neoaorta, laceration of the right coronary artery, and congenital stenosis of the coronary sinus involving its termination. In most patients with coronary insufficiency, death occurred within the first day after completion of the operation, and most of these patients had acute myocardial infarction. The second most common cause of death identified in this series was excessive pulmonary blood flow. Central shunts were more prevalent than modified Blalock-Taussig shunts in the patients who were believed to have died of pulmonary overcirculation. Obstruction to pulmonary blood flow was identified as the third most common cause of death in this series. Acute thrombosis of the modified Blalock-Taussig shunt was identified in 14 patients. This was variously attributed to stenosis of the superior stoma, stenosis of the inferior stoma, excessive length of the shunt, anastomotic stricture, and acute low cardiac output. The authors speculated that small shunts may be associated with an increased risk of thrombosis. Obstruction of the neoaortic arch was found in 17 patients. In several cases, this was produced by kinking and inward bulging of the patch used to augment the aorta. In most instances, the stenosis was found at the distal end of the transverse arch. Other potential causes of death identified in the series included right ventricular failure, bleeding, infection, tricuspid or common atrial ventricular valve dysfunction, enterocolitis, and sudden death presumed to be related to arrhythmias. In 26 patients (21%), more than one factor was identified and was thought to be involved in the cause of death.

COMPLICATIONS AND LATE CONSIDERATIONS
AORTIC ARCH OBSTRUCTION

As part of the analysis of surgical experience at The Children's Hospital of Philadelphia, serial echocardiograms were reviewed to assess growth of the reconstructed aorta. In a group of 50 patients, measurements were made from echocardiograms performed immediately after the Norwood stage 1 palliation and at 2 later points (1-11 years of age). Growth in diameter of the transverse arch paralleled that seen in the normal population. In addition, autopsy specimens were evaluated in a group of 10 patients who had died 12 to 34 months after Norwood stage 1 palliation. There was a mean increase in width of the native aortic tissue of 0.67 cm ($P <$ .01), with no significant change in homograft circumference. Thus, Mahle et al[59] concluded that the reconstructed aorta increased its size in a fashion that paralleled that seen in the normal population, and the size increase was attributable to growth of native aortic tissue.

Fraisse et al[60] undertook a study looking at aortic arch obstruction after the stage 1 Norwood procedure. This investigation revealed that aortic arch obstruction generally develops within 6 months of the stage 1 procedure, with a probability of 21%. Very few patients develop obstruction beyond 6 months. Patients who develop aortic arch obstruction showed evidence of moderate-to-severe tricuspid regurgitation and abnormal abdominal aortic Doppler flow patterns. After the first 30 days after stage 1 palliation, the risk of death was higher in patients who developed aortic arch obstruction than in those that did not. Sensitivity of echocardiography in detecting this lesion was only 73%, with a specificity of 92%. In view of the increased risk of death associated with aortic arch obstruction, the authors concluded that early cardiac catheterization with possible intervention should be considered in those patients who show evidence of right ventricular dysfunction, tricuspid regurgitation, or abnormal abdominal aortic Doppler flow patterns. This report and others, have confirmed that in the most instances, aortic arch obstructions can be dealt with successfully by balloon angioplasty in the catheterization laboratory.

FATE OF THE PULMONIC VALVE IN THE SYSTEMIC CIRCULATION

The function and durability of the pulmonary valve in the systemic circulation after aortopulmonary anastomosis has long been a concern. Chin et al[61] used color Doppler flow mapping to examine 45 patients with pulmonary artery to ascending aortic anastomosis at a median of 202 days postoperatively. Most of these patients had HLHS. Mild pulmonary valve regurgitation was noted in 24% and moderate regurgitation in 3%. In this study, maximum follow-up was 2.8 years. Progression of pulmonary valve regurgitation from mild or moderate to a severe level is rare. In at least one instance, this has been managed by replacement of the neoaortic valve (pulmonary valve) with a prosthesis, more than a year after the Fontan procedure (Jacobs, personal communication).

NEUROLOGIC AND DEVELOPMENTAL OUTCOME

Mahle et al[62] performed a follow-up survey on 115 children aged 9.0 ± 2.0 years who had undergone staged reconstructive surgery for HLHS at The Children's Hospital of Philadelphia. The parents of the majority of patients described academic performance as average (42%) or above average (42%), with one third of children receiving some form of special education. Standardized cognitive testing of a subgroup of 28 patients (followed locally) aged 8.6 ± 2 years, demonstrated a median full scale IQ of 86 (50-116). Multivariate analysis demonstrated that a history of preoperative seizures predicted lower full-scale IQ. Kern et al[63] reported an investigation of 14 children with HLHS older than 3 years who had undergone at least 2 surgical stages at Columbia Presbyterian Medical Center. IQ testing was performed on these children, and the results were compared with those of 10 family controls. They were also tested for adaptive behavior. Median scores for full-scale IQ and adaptive behavior were 88 and 91, respectively, with normal values being 100 ± 15. A negative correlation was found between the stage 1 circulatory arrest time and the full-scale IQ.

They concluded that children with HLHS usually function in the low-normal range for intelligence and adaptive behavior.

CORONARY PERFUSION

Donnelly et al[64] evaluated coronary blood flow in infants after repair of congenital heart malformations. Five infants who had undergone Norwood stage 1 palliation for HLHS were compared with 5 patients who had undergone biventricular repair of other types of heart malformations. Positron emission tomography was used to estimate coronary blood flow. In the biventricular group, resting coronary flow in the left ventricle was estimated at 1.8 ± 0.2 mL/min per gram, compared with 1.0 ± 0.3 mL/min per gram for the HLHS group. The authors concluded that infants with repaired heart disease have higher resting coronary blood flow and less coronary flow reserve than the levels previously reported for adults. After the Norwood stage 1 palliation, infants have less indexed coronary blood flow to the systemic ventricle than do infants with biventricular circulation. It was inferred that this phenomenon may contribute to the overall risk of mortality at the time of, and after stage 1 palliation for HLHS.

Fogel et al[65] used transesophageal echocardiography and Doppler flow estimates to assess coronary blood flow in patients with aortic atresia. After stage 1 palliation, coronary blood flow was predominantly during systole. After the hemi-Fontan procedure, the pattern of coronary blood flow was changed, with a marked increase in flow during diastole (as in normal patients). Quantitative estimation of coronary blood flow after stage 1 palliation and after the hemi-Fontan, revealed considerably higher values after stage 1 palliation (982 ± 322 vs 589 ± 334 mL/min per square meter). The velocity time integral and peak flow velocity were also found to be higher after stage 1 palliation. The authors inferred that this was related to the increased energy demands of the systemic ventricle pumping both systemic and pulmonary blood flow. These parameters were all decreased after the hemi-Fontan procedure.

EXERCISE PERFORMANCE

Exercise performance of patients with a Fontan-type connection has been assessed by numerous investigators. Joshi et al[66] compared patients with HLHS who had undergone a Fontan procedure, with a second group of Fontan patients with a systemic right ventricle (non-HLHS) and a third group with a systemic left ventricle. They were evaluated for resting pulmonary mechanics followed by maximal exercise testing with a bicycle or treadmill protocol. No significant differences were seen between the HLHS group and the comparison groups for the following parameters: maximal heart rate, maximal oxygen consumption, respiratory exchange ratio, breathing reserve, and arterial oxygen saturation at rest or during exercise. The authors concluded that exercise performance for patients with total cavopulmonary type of Fontan connection was comparable, independent of ventricular morphology or specific diagnosis.

CONCLUSION

Since the pioneering efforts 2 decades ago of Norwood and others, standardization and widespread acceptance of techniques for staged reconstructive surgical management of HLHS have brought us to a period of steadily decreasing mortality for what was once considered a uniformly fatal disease. Clearly, the greatest surgical challenge is the palliative management of neonates with duct-dependent systemic circulation and a diminutive ascending aorta. Interval attrition between initial palliation and the eventual second-stage surgical procedure remains another significant problem. This may in part be related to the abnormal physiology of coronary perfusion that exists in the palliated state, but is also impacted by such complications as aortic arch obstruction. Mortality at the time of the hemi-Fontan procedure is relatively rare (5%-10%), and the interposition of this intermediate operation has had an important positive impact on survival from the eventual completion Fontan procedure.

Technical advances are currently being made both with respect to preoperative, intraoperative, and postoperative management of the abnormal physiologic state of these patients, and with respect to the surgical exercises themselves. In the latter area, modifications to operative techniques are still evolving, with a goal of reducing the potential harmful effects of cardiopulmonary bypass and hypothermic circulatory arrest. Further progress in these areas is expected to contribute to the optimization not only of survival, but of functional and neurologic outcomes. Growth of the surgically created pathways remains a consideration and is the subject of ongoing investigations. The lessons learned in the surgical management of HLHS have not only impacted dramatically on the lives of children with this common and serious congenital heart malformation, but have contributed immensely to the successful management of the entire spectrum of critical heart malformations requiring surgical intervention very early in life.

REFERENCES

1. Lev M: Pathologic anatomy and interrelationship of hypoplasia of the aortic tract complexes. *Lab Invest* 1:61, 1952.
2. Noonan JA, Nadas AS: The hypoplastic left heart syndrome: An analysis of 101 cases. *Pediatr Clin North Am* 5:1029-1056, 1958.
3. Bharati S, Lev M: The surgical anatomy of hypoplasia of aortic tract complex. *J Thorac Cardiovasc Surg* 88:97-101, 1984.
4. Jacobs ML, Blackstone EH, Bailey LL: Intermediate survival in neonates with aortic atresia: A multi-institutional study. *J Thorac Cardiovasc Surg* 417-431, 1998.
5. Reis PM, Punch MR, van de Ven CJM: Obstetric management of 219 infants with hypoplastic left heart syndrome. *Obstet Gynecol* 179:1150-1154, 1998.
6. Rychik J, Rome JJ, Collins MH, et al: The hypoplastic left heart syndrome with intact atrial septum: Atrial morphology, pulmonary vascular histopathology and outcome. *J Am Coll Cardiol* 34:554-560, 1999.
7. Chang AC, Huhta JC, Yoon GY, et al: Diagnosis, transport, and outcome in fetuses with left ventricular outflow tract obstruction. *J Thorac Cardiovasc Surg* 102:841-848, 1991.
8. Atz AM, Feinstein JA, Jonas RA, et al: Preoperative management of pulmonary venous hypertension in hypoplastic left heart syndrome with restrictive atrial septal defect. *Am J Cardiol* 83:1224-1228, 1999.
9. Kumar RK, Newburger JW, Gauvreau K, et al: Comparison of outcome when hypoplastic left heart syndrome and transposition of the great arteries are diagnosed prenatally versus when diagnosis of these two conditions is made only postnatally. *Am J Cardiol* 83:1649-1653, 1999.
10. Cayler GG, Smeloff EA, Miller GE Jr: Surgical palliation of hypoplastic left side of the heart. *N Engl J Med* 282:780-783, 1970.
11. Freedom RM, Cullham JAG, Rowe RD: Aortic atresia with normal left ventricle: Distinctive angiocardiographic findings. *Cathet Cardiovasc Diagn* 3:283-295, 1977.
12. Litwin SB, Van Praagh R, Bernhard WF: A palliative operation for certain infants with aortic arch interruption. *Ann Thorac Surg* 14:369-375, 1972.
13. Albert HM, Bryant LR: A proposed technique for treatment of hypoplastic left heart syndrome. *J Cardiovasc Surg (Torino)* 19:257, 1978.
14. Mohri H, Horiuchi T, Haneda K, et al: Surgical treatment for hypoplastic left heart syndrome: Case reports. *J Thorac Cardiovasc Surg* 78:223-228, 1979.
15. Doty DB, Knotts HW: Hypoplastic left heart syndrome: Experience with an operation to establish functionally normal circulation. *J Thorac Cardiovasc Surg* 74:624-630, 1977.
16. Norwood WI, Kirklin JK, Sanders SP: Hypoplastic left heart syndrome: Experience with palliative surgery. *Am J Cardiol* 45:87-91, 1980.
17. Doty DB, Marwin WJ Jr, Schieken RM, et al: Hypoplastic left heart syndrome: Successful palliation with a new operation. *J Thorac Cardiovasc Surg* 80:148-152, 1980.

18. Levitsky S, Van Der Horst RL, Hastreiter AR, et al: *J Thorac Cardiovasc Surg* 79:456-461, 1980.
19. Norwood WI, Lang P, Hansen DD: Physiologic repair of aortic atresia–hypoplastic left heart syndrome. *N Engl J Med* 308:23-26, 1983.
20. Pigott JD, Murphy JD, Barber G, et al: Palliative reconstructive surgery for hypoplastic left heart syndrome. *Ann Thorac Surg* 45:122-128, 1988.
21. Jacobs ML, Rychik J, Rome J, et al: Early reduction of the volume work of the single ventricle: The hemi-Fontan operation. *Ann Thorac Surg* 62:456, 1996.
22. Jacobs ML, Norwood WI Jr: Fontan operation: Influence of modifications on morbidity and mortality. *Ann Thorac Surg* 58:945-952, 1994.
23. Jacobs ML: Hypoplastic left heart syndrome, in Kaiser LR, Kron IL, Spray TS (eds): *Mastery of Cardiothoracic Surgery*. Philadelphia, Lippincott-Raven, 1998, pp 857-866.
24. Tam VKH, Miller BE, Murphy K: Modified Fontan without use of cardiopulmonary bypass. *Ann Thorac Surg* 68:1698-1704, 1999.
25. Hickey PR: Neurological sequelae associated with deep hypothermia circulatory arrest. *Ann Thorac Surg* 65:65S-70S, 1998.
26. Jonas RA, Wernovsky G, Ware J, et al: The Boston Circulatory Arrest Study: Perioperative neurologic and developmental outcome after the arterial switch operation. *Circulation* 86:I-360, 1992.
27. Glauser TA, Rorke LB, Weinberg PM, et al: Acquired neuropathologic lesions associated with the hypoplastic left heart syndrome. *Pediatrics* 85:991-1000, 1990.
28. Fraser CD Jr, Mee RBB: Modified Norwood procedure for hypoplastic left heart syndrome. *Ann Thorac Surg* 60:546S-549S, 1995.
29. Asou T, Kado H, Imoto Y, et al: Selective cerebral perfusion technique during aortic arch repair in neonates. *Ann Thorac Surg* 61:1546-1548, 1996.
30. Pigula FA, Siewers RD, Nemoto EM: Regional perfusion of the brain during neonatal arch reconstruction. *J Thorac Cardiovasc Surg* 117:1023-1024, 1999.
31. Swain JA, McDonald TJ, Griffith PK, et al: Low flow hypothermic cardiopulmonary bypass protects the brain. *J Thorac Cardiovasc Surg* 192:76-83, 1991.
32. McElhinney DB, Reddy VM, Silverman NH, et al: Modified Damus-Kaye-Stansel procedure for single ventricle, subaortic stenosis, and arch obstruction in neonates and infants: Midterm results and techniques for avoiding circulatory arrest. *J Thorac Cardiovasc Surg* 114:718-726, 1997.
33. Kishimoto H, Kawahira Y, Mori T, et al: The modified Norwood palliation on a beating heart. *J Thorac Cardiovasc Surg* 118:1130-1132, 1999.
34. Imoto Y, Kado H, Yasui H, et al: Norwood procedure without circulatory arrest. *J Thorac Cardiovasc Surg* 68:559-561, 1999.
35. Ishino K, Stumper O, Brawn WJ, et al: The modified Norwood procedure for hypoplastic left heart syndrome: Early to intermediate results of 120 patients with particular reference to aortic arch repair. *J Thorac Cardiovasc Surg* 117:920-930, 1999.

36. Pridjian AK, Culpepper WC, McGettisan M, et al: Early results with a new procedure for hypoplastic left heart syndrome and aortic atresia. *J La State Med Soc* 147:308-312, 1995.

37. Schmid FX, Kampmann C, Oelert H, et al: Adjustable tourniquet to manipulate pulmonary blood flow after Norwood operations. *Ann Thorac Surg* 68:2306-2309, 1999.

38. Jacobs ML, Murphy JD, Nicolson SC, et al: Manipulation of inspired carbon dioxide in neonates with one ventricle and systemic to pulmonary artery shunt. *Circulation* 84:238, 1991.

39. Morray JP, Lynn AM, Mansfield PB: Effect of pH and $PaCO_2$ on pulmonary and systemic hemodynamics after surgery in children with congenital heart disease and pulmonary hypertension. *J Pediatr* 113:474-479, 1988.

40. Gullquist SD, Schmitz ML, Hannon GD, et al: Carbon dioxide in the inspired gas improves early postoperative survival in neonates with congenital heart disease following stage I palliation (Norwood). *Circulation* 86:I-360S, 1992.

41. Mora GA, Pizarro C, Jacobs ML, et al: Experimental model of single ventricle: Influence of carbon dioxide on pulmonary vascular dynamics. *Circulation* 90:II-43-II-46, 1994.

42. Reddy VM, Liddicoat JR, Fineman JR, et al: Fetal model of single ventricle physiology: Hemodynamic effects of oxygen, carbon dioxide, and hypoxia in the early postnatal period. *J Thorac Cardiovasc Surg* 112:437-449, 1996.

43. Barnea O, Santamore WP, Ross A, et al: Estimation of oxygen delivery in newborns with a univentricular circulation. *Circulation* 98:1407-1413, 1998.

44. Tweddell JS, Hoffman GM, Kessel MW, et al: Phenoxybenzamine improves systemic oxygen delivery after the Norwood procedure. *Ann Thorac Surg* 67:161-168, 1999.

45. Day RW, Barton AJ, Pysher TJ, et al: Pulmonary vascular resistance of children treated with nitrogen during early infancy. *Ann Thorac Surg* 65:1400-1404, 1998.

46. Kirklin JW, Barratt-Boyes BG: Hypothermia, circulatory arrest, and cardiopulmonary bypass, in Kirklin JW, Barratt-Boyes BG (eds): *Cardiac Surgery*, ed 2. New York, John Wiley & Sons, 1993, p 74.

47. Tchervenkov CI, Thata SA, Jutras LC, et al: Biventricular repair in neonates with hypoplastic left heart complex. *Ann Thorac Surg* 66:1350-1357, 1998.

48. Rhodes LA, Colan SD, Perry SB, et al: Predictors of survival in neonates with critical aortic stenosis. *Circulation* 84:2325-2335, 1991.

49. Keane JF, Norwood WI, Bernhard WF: Surgery for aortic stenosis in infancy. *Circulation* 68:182, 1982.

50. Karl TR, Sano S, Brawn WJ, et al: Critical aortic stenosis in the first month of life: Surgical results in 26 infants. *Ann Thorac Surg* 50:105-109, 1990.

51. Reddy VM, McElhinney DB, Hanley FL: Ross procedure in children. *Isr J Med Sci* 32:888-891, 1996.

52. Serraf A, Piot JD, Bonnet N, et al: Biventricular repair approach in ductal-dependent neonates with hypoplastic but morphologically normal left ventricle. *J Am Coll Cardiol* 33:827-834, 1999.

53. Tani LY, Minich LL, Pagotto LT, et al: Left heart hypoplasia and neonatal aortic arch obstruction: Is the Rhodes left ventricular adequacy score applicable? *J Thorac Cardiovasc Surg* 118:81-86, 1999.

54. Minich LL, Tani LY, Hawkins JA, et al: Possibility of post natal left ventricular growth in selected infants with non apex forming left ventricles. *Am Heart J* 133:570, 1997.

55. Reyes A II, Bove EL, Mosca RS, et al: Tricuspid valve repair in children with hypoplastic left heart syndrome during staged surgical reconstruction. *Circulation* 96:II-341S–II-345S, 1997.

56. Forbess JM, Cook N, Roth SJ, et al: Ten-year institutional experience with palliative surgery or hypoplastic left heart syndrome: Risk factors related to stage I mortality. *Circulation* 92:II-262S–II-266S, 1995.

57. Daebritz SH, Nollert GDA, Zurakowski D, et al: Results of Norwood stage I operation: Comparison of hypoplastic left heart syndrome with other malformations. *J Thorac Cardiovasc Surg* 199:358-367, 2000.

58. Bartrum U, Grünenfelder J, Van Praagh R: Causes of death after the modified Norwood procedure: A study of 122 postmortem cases. *Ann Thorac Surg* 64:1795-1802, 1997.

59. Mahle WT, Rychik J, Weinber PM, et al: Growth characteristics of the aortic arch after the Norwood operation. *J Am Coll Cardiol* 32:1951-1954, 1998.

60. Fraisse A, Colan SD, Jonas RA, et al: Accuracy of echocardiography for detection of aortic arch obstruction after stage I Norwood procedure. *Am Heart J* 135:230-236, 1998.

61. Chin AJ, Barber G, Helton JG, et al: Fate of the pulmonic valve after proximal pulmonary artery-to-ascending aorta anastomosis for aortic outflow obstruction. *Am J Cardiol* 62:435-438, 1988.

62. Mahle WT, Clancy RR, Moss EM, et al: Neurodevelopmental outcome and lifestyle assessment in school-aged and adolescent children with hypoplastic left heart syndrome. *Pediatrics* 105:1082-1089, 2000.

63. Kern JH, Hinton VJ, Nereo NE, et al: Early developmental outcome after the Norwood procedure for hypoplastic left heart syndrome. *Pediatrics* 102:1148-1152, 1998.

64. Donnelly JP, Bove EL, Kulik TJ, et al: Resting coronary flow reserve in human infants after repair or palliation of congenital heart defects as measured by positron emission tomography. *J Thorac Cardiovasc Surg* 115:103-110, 1998.

65. Fogel MA, Rychik J, Vetter J, et al: Effect of volume unloading surgery on coronary flow dynamics in patients with aortic atresia. *J Thorac Cardiovasc Surg* 113:718-727, 1997.

66. Joshi VM, Carey A, Simpson P, et al:. Exercise performance following repair of hypoplastic left heart syndrome: A comparison with other types of Fontan patients. *Pediatr Cardiol* 18:357-360, 1997.

CHAPTER 3

Aortic Surgery in the Marfan Syndrome

Tirone E. David, MD
Professor of Surgery, University of Toronto, and Chief, Division of
Cardiovascular Surgery, Toronto General Hospital, Toronto, Ontario,
Canada

The Marfan syndrome is a relatively common (affecting approximately 1 in 10,000 individuals) autosomal dominant disorder that occurs in all races and ethnic groups. It is caused by mutations in the gene that encodes fibrillin-1 (FBN1) on chromosome 15. This is a large gene (approximately 10,000 nucleotides in the mRNA); thus, identification of mutation is a complex task. For this reason, the diagnosis of the Marfan syndrome remains largely a clinical one. In view of the classic phenotype of the Marfan syndrome, failure to diagnose appears surprising, but marked clinical variability, age dependence of all its manifestations, and a high rate of new mutation make the detection of mildly affected, sporadic cases difficult. Current criteria depend on a family history and manifestations in the eyes, the skeleton, and the cardiovascular system. Clinically, 2 of 3 systems must be affected for the syndrome to be diagnosed. The presence of manifestations such as aortic root dilation, aortic dissection in a nonhypertensive young patient, ectopia lentis, and dura ectasia, is more important diagnostically than features common in other connective tissue disorders such as scoliosis, joint hypermobility, myopia and mitral valve prolapse.

The most common cardiovascular features are mitral valve prolapse and dilation of the aortic sinuses. These anatomical abnormalities may cause mitral regurgitation, aortic regurgitation and aortic dissection, which, if untreated, are the usual causes of death for patients with the Marfan syndrome.

Mitral valve prolapse is age dependent and more common in women. It is present in 60% to 80% of patients as seen with echocardiography, but only one fourth will have mitral regurgitation develop. The mitral annulus is often dilated and may attain large sizes, particularly when mitral regurgitation is present. The mitral annulus may become heavily calcified and occasionally have the "horseshoe" appearance.

The dilation of the aortic root is often progressive. The rate of increase, which varies somewhat, is usually less than 1 or 2 mm per year. If the diameter of the aortic root is less than 1.5 times of the predicted diameter for the body surface area, annual measurements with echocardiography are sufficient. When the diameter exceeds 40 mm, biannual studies are warranted. Acute aortic dissection is rare in patients with aortic root aneurysm of less than 50 mm, unless they have family history of aortic dissection. The dissection in most patients starts at the level of the sinotubular junction (type A aortic dissection). In approximately 10% of the patients it starts just beyond the left subclavian artery (type B aortic dissection). Not all patients with acute dissection experience severe chest pain. For this reason, a high degree of suspicion is important to diagnose dissection in these patients.

Patients with the Marfan syndrome should be followed up at regular intervals. Doppler echocardiography is the best diagnostic tool for monitoring changes in the mitral valve and in the aortic root. Magnetic resonance images of the remaining thoracic and abdominal aorta should also be obtained when indicated. Beta-blockage has been shown to be effective in reducing the rate of aortic root dilation.[1]

Pregnancy in women with the Marfan syndrome has 2 potential problems: (1) the risk of having a child who will inherit the disorder and (2) acute aortic dissection during the third trimester, parturition, or the first month postpartum. There is a 50% risk of inheriting the syndrome. The risk of acute aortic dissection is less known, but it appears to be very low in patients in whom the diameter of the aortic root does not exceed 40 mm and cardiac function is normal.[2]

INDICATIONS FOR SURGERY
MITRAL REGURGITATION

Patients with symptomatic mitral regurgitation should be operated on. Those with asymptomatic mitral regurgitation should also be operated on if transesophageal echocardiography suggests that mitral valve repair is feasible. Heavily calcified posterior mitral annulus ("horseshoe" appearance), mitral annulus diameter greater than 50 mm, severe prolapse of the anterior leaflet, calcified papillary muscle and calcified chordae tendineae to the anterior leaflet make valve repair more difficult and the long-term results are less predictable.[3,4] Dilation of the posterior mitral annulus is largely caused by partial detachment of the fibrous annulus from the ventricular wall, and this lesion is correctable by means of mitral valvuloplasty.

AORTIC ROOT DILATION

Dilation of the aortic root is the principal indication for elective operation in patients with the Marfan syndrome. Traditionally, surgery is indicated when the diameter of the aortic root exceeds 55 mm.[5,6] For patients with a family history of aortic dissection, surgery should be performed when the diameter of the aortic root approaches 50 mm.[5,6] Elective surgery should be recommended earlier if transesophageal echocardiography shows normal aortic valve cusps because the feasibility of an aortic valve–sparing operation decreases as the diameter of the aortic root increases.[7,8] Our experience indicates that practically all patients with the Marfan syndrome can have an aortic valve–sparing procedure when the diameter of the aortic root is less than 55 mm.[7,8] The probability of preserving the aortic valve decreases as the diameter of the aortic root increases. The diameter of the sinotubular junction is even more important than the diameter of the aortic sinuses in predicting reparability of the aortic valve.[7,8] Isolated dilation of the aortic sinuses does not cause aortic valve dysfunction[9]; however, as the sinotubular junction or aortic annulus dilate, the mechanical stress on aortic cusps is increased and they become thinner, overstretched, and develop stress fenestrations along the commissural areas.[8] We believe that elective surgery should be performed when the aortic root approaches 50 mm, or even less if the patient has aortic insufficiency or a family history of aortic dissection, as long as an aortic valve–sparing operation is deemed feasible.

AORTIC INSUFFICIENCY

Aortic insufficiency is often caused by dilation of the sinotubular junction or the aortic annulus, or both. As the sinotubular junction dilates, the aortic cusps are pulled away from the center of the aortic root, and central aortic insufficiency ensues. If this is left untreated, the cusps become damaged and the severity of aortic insufficiency increases. Transesophageal Doppler echocardiography often shows multiple jets of aortic insufficiency in these more advanced stages of valve dysfunction. If the aortic insufficiency is caused by dilation of the sinotubular junction, surgery is usually dictated by the size of the aortic root. If it is due to diseased cusps and the aortic root is not dilated (a rare situation), operation is dictated by changes in ventricular function or symptoms. Occasionally, a patient with the Marfan syndrome has a bicuspid aortic valve and one of the cusps may prolapse and cause aortic insufficiency before dilation of the sinotubular junction becomes evident.

AORTIC DISSECTION

Patients with acute type A aortic dissection should be treated with immediate surgery. Patients with chronic type A aortic dissection should be operated on when the diameter of the aortic root approaches 50 mm or when the diameter of the false lumen anywhere in the thoracic aorta exceeds 50 mm. Type B aortic dissection in patients with the Marfan syndrome is treated conservatively with β-blockers, blood pressure control, and close observation. It has been our experience that extension of the dissection and more rapid expansion of the false lumen are far more common in patients with the Marfan syndrome than in those without it. Thus, replacement of the thoracic and abdominal aorta is often needed for these patients.

SURGICAL TREATMENT OF AORTIC ROOT ANEURYSM
CHOICE OF OPERATIVE PROCEDURE

The standard treatment for patients with aortic root aneurysm has been composite replacement of the aortic valve and ascending aorta with a biological or mechanical valved conduit.[5,6] During the past decade, however, there has been an increased interest in preserving the aortic valve in these patients. The experience accumulated thus far justifies the continued use of aortic valve–sparing operations in patients with the Marfan syndrome.[7,8,10,11] Although it is possible to predict with high accuracy, by means of transesophageal echocardiography, which patients are candidates for aortic valve sparing, the final decision is always made after careful inspection of the aortic valve cusps. They must be normal or near normal to be preserved in patients with the Marfan syndrome.[12,13] If the aortic cusps are normal, reimplantation of the aortic valve or remodeling of the aortic root should be performed. We believe that the first procedure is the best for patients with the Marfan syndrome. These aortic valve–sparing operations must be performed with the use of transesophageal echocardiography. If the cusps are thinned, overstretched, or contain multiple fenestrations, aortic root replacement should be performed. It can be done with an aortic valve homograft or a tubular Dacron graft containing a mechanical or a bioprosthetic heart valve.[14]

AORTIC ROOT REMODELING

After the aortic cusps have been inspected and found to be normal or to contain minimal abnormalities, the 3 aortic sinuses are excised, leaving 4 to 5 mm of arterial wall attached to the aortic annulus and around each coronary artery, as illustrated in Fig 1. We believe that an aortic annuloplasty is necessary in patients with the Marfan syndrome with or without annuloaortic ectasia because of the progressive nature of this disorder. Thus, a band of Dacron fabric should be secured on the outside of the fibrous component of the left ventricular outflow tract at the lowest level of aortic annulus, as illustrated in Fig 2. Multiple horizontal mattress sutures of 3-0 or 4-0 polyester are passed from the inside to the outside of the left ventricular outflow tract through a single hori-

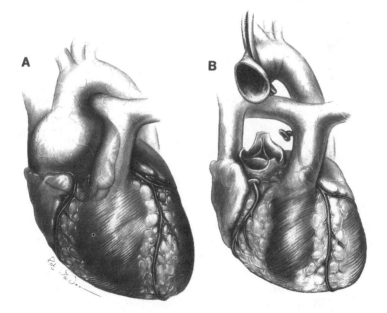

FIGURE 1.
Aortic valve sparing: the 3 aortic sinuses are excised, leaving 4 to 5 mm of arterial wall attached to the aortic annulus. (From David TE: Remodeling the aortic root and preservation of the native aortic valve. *Op Tech Cardiac Thorac Surg* 1:44-56, 1996. Used with permission.)

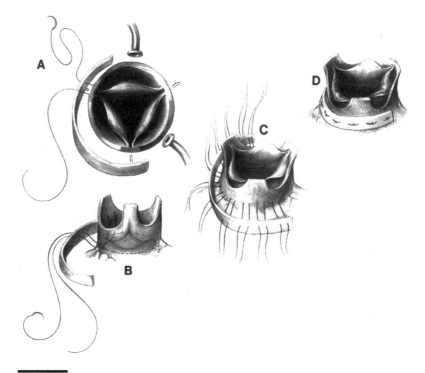

FIGURE 2.
Aortic annuloplasty during remodeling of the aortic root: the fibrous component of the left ventricular outflow tract immediately beneath the aortic annulus is reinforced with a band of Dacron graft. The sutures are placed along a single horizontal plane. (From David TE: Remodeling the aortic root and preservation of the native aortic valve. *Op Tech Cardiac Thorac Surg* 1:44-56, 1996. Used with permission.)

zontal plane immediately below the level of the aortic annulus. If reduction of the annulus is needed, it should be done beneath the commissures of the non-coronary cusp. The diameter of the aortic annulus must not exceed the average length of the free margins of the aortic cusps.

A tubular Dacron graft of a diameter equal to the average length of the free margins of the aortic cusps is selected. One of its ends is divided into 3 equal parts, and longitudinal cuts of lengths equal to the diameter of the graft are made, as shown in Fig 3. The 3 commissures of the aortic valve are suspended into the tailored graft with horizontal mattress sutures of 4-0 polypropylene. The graft should lie on the inside of the remnants of the aortic sinuses. These sutures are then used to secure the neo-aortic sinus of

Dacron to the aortic annulus in a continuous fashion. The coronary arteries are reimplanted into their respective neo-aortic sinuses, as illustrated in Fig 4. The distal portion of the graft is anastomosed to the distal ascending aorta or the transverse arch graft if the arch was also replaced.

REIMPLANTATION OF THE AORTIC VALVE

The excision of the aortic sinuses is performed as described above, but more arterial wall is left in the lower part of the aortic annulus than along the commissural areas. We normally leave 3 to 5 mm of sinus wall along the commissural areas and 6 to 8 mm in the lower

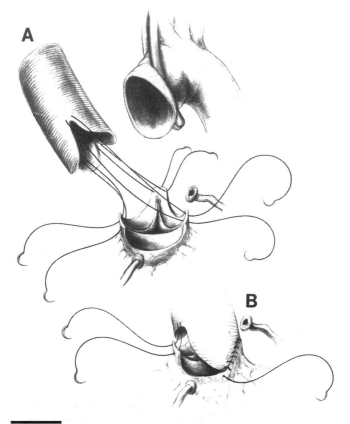

FIGURE 3.
Remodeling of the aortic root: a tailored tubular Dacron graft is used to create neo-aortic sinuses by suturing it to the aortic annulus and remnants of the aortic sinuses. (From David TE: Remodeling the aortic root and preservation of the native aortic valve. *Op Tech Cardiac Thorac Surg* 1:44-56, 1996. Used with permission.)

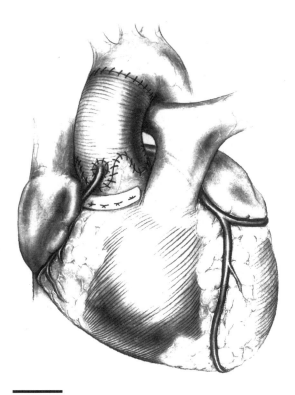

FIGURE 4.
Remodeling of the aortic root: the coronary arteries are reimplanted into their respective neo-aortic sinuses. (From David TE: Remodeling the aortic root and preservation of the native aortic valve. *Op Tech Cardiac Thorac Surg* 1:44-56, 1996. Used with permission).

part of the sinuses, as illustrated in Fig 1. The coronary arteries are detached from their sinuses, leaving 4 to 5 mm of arterial wall around them. Next, multiple horizontal mattress sutures of 3-0 or 4-0 polyester are passed from the inside to the outside of the left ventricular outflow tract through a single horizontal plane along its fibrous components and immediately below the aortic annulus along its muscular component, as illustrated in Fig 5. Ten to 12 sutures are usually needed. Next, the length of the free margin of each cusp is measured by gently pulling the commissures apart. A tubular Dacron 4-mm larger in diameter than the average lengths of the free margins of the aortic cusps is selected. One of its ends is divided in equidistant thirds to correspond to the commissures of the aortic valve. A 1-cm triangular resection is made in one of the thirds to correspond to the commissure between the right and left aortic cusps, as illustrated in Fig 5. The polyester sutures passed through the left ventricular outflow tract are now passed from the inside to the outside of the tailored end of the Dacron graft. It is important to distribute these sutures equidistantly in the graft. If the aortic annulus was larger than the graft, plication of annulus should occur only beneath the commissures of the non-coronary cusp, which are made entirely of fibrous tissue. By gently pulling on all sutures, the aortic valve will be placed on the inside of the graft. All sutures are then tied on the outside of the graft. Care must be exercised to avoid causing a purse-string of the aortic annulus. The graft is cut 5 or 6 cm in length, and both the graft and

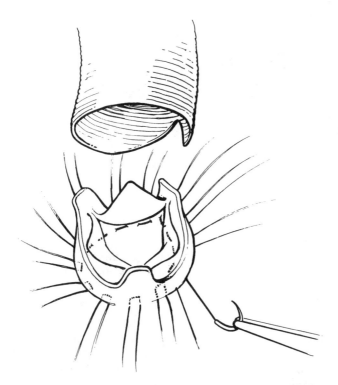

FIGURE 5.
Reimplantation of the aortic valve: multiple horizontal mattress sutures are placed from the inside to the outside of the left ventricular outflow tract. These sutures are placed on a single horizontal plane along the fibrous components of the left ventricular outflow tract and they follow the scalloped shape of the aortic annulus along the muscular interventricular septum. The tubular Dacron graft is also scalloped along the commissure between the left and right cusps.

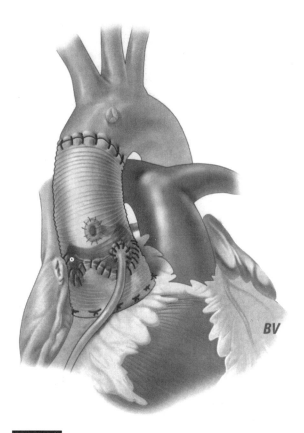

FIGURE 6.
Reimplantation of the aortic valve: the 3 commissures are resuspended inside the Dacron graft and the remnants of the aortic sinuses are sutured to the Dacron with a continuous 4-0 polypropylene. The coronary arteries are reimplanted into their respective neoaortic sinuses.

the 3 commissures are gently pulled upward. Horizontal mattress 4-0 polypropylene sutures with a pledget are used to secure the upper part of commissure on the Dacron graft. The valve is then tested by injecting saline solution into the graft and observing the coaptation of the cusp. If the commissures are correctly aligned, the polypropylene sutures are tied on the outside of the graft. These sutures are then used to secure the remnants of the aortic sinuses to the Dacron graft. This layer of suture must be carefully done because it has to be hemostatic. The coronary arteries are reimplanted in their respective sinuses, as illustrated in Fig 6. Bulging neoaortic sinuses can be created by plicating the spaces between the commissures of the valve at the sinotubular junction. These plications should be of approximately 4 mm each. This is equivalent to a reduction of 4 mm in diameter of the sinotubular junction.

SURGERY FOR TYPE A AORTIC DISSECTION

Patients with acute type A aortic dissection should be treated with immediate surgery. Cardiopulmonary bypass is established by cannulating the right atrium and a peripheral artery (femoral or axillary). We firmly believe that aortic clamping should be avoided before repair of the aneurysm in these patients—particularly if the arterial return is through a femoral artery.[15] The patient should be cooled and the circulation arrested. We routinely use cold retrograde cerebral perfusion during circulatory arrest. The ascending aorta should be transected just before the innominate artery and just above the sinotubular junction. Most intimal tears in patients with the Marfan syndrome start at the level of, or immediately above, the sinotubular junction. The aortic arch is explored. If there it is not dilated and there are no intimal tears in the transverse arch or proximal descending thoracic aorta, we suture a tubular Dacron graft at the level of the origin of the innominate artery with continuous suture of 4-0 polypropylene in a fine needle. The graft should lie on the inside of the true lumen. If the transverse arch is dilated or contains intimal tears, we perform complete arch replacement. The elephant trunk technique can be used if the descending aorta is dilated, but often the true lumen is too small to allow a graft of adequate diameter into it. Thus, a simple end-to-end anastomosis between the graft and the proximal descending thoracic aorta is effected and the brachiocephalic vessels are reimplanted with a small amount of aortic wall around them either as an island or separately, depending on the local pathology. If a femoral artery had been used for arterial return, the cannula is removed from the femoral artery and inserted into the graft for antegrade perfusion. If an axillary artery was used for arterial return, it need not be changed. Cardiopulmonary bypass is reestablished, and the aortic root is dealt with as the patient is rewarmed.

The aortic sinuses of patients with the Marfan syndrome must be replaced. Either an aortic valve–sparing operation or a valved conduit should be used to repair the aortic root.

COMPOSITE REPLACEMENT OF THE AORTIC VALVE AND ASCENDING AORTA

If the aortic valve cusps are abnormal, replacement of the aortic valve and sinuses is performed with a valved conduit. This can be a commercially available tubular Dacron graft containing a mechanical valve, a stentless biological valve such as aortic homo-graft or the Medtronic Freestyle porcine aortic root (Medtronic, Minneapolis, Minn), or a bioprosthetic valve inside a tubular Dacron graft, which can be prepared in the operating room.

The aortic root need not be dissected circumferentially, as in an aortic valve–sparing procedure, but the coronary arteries should be detached from their sinuses and mobilized to allow for a tension-free reimplantation in the aortic graft. The right coronary artery is usually more displaced than the left, and care must be exercised during its reimplantation to prevent kinking. When a mechanical valve is used, the conduit should be secured to the aortic annulus by using inverting horizontal mattress sutures with Teflon pledgets on the outside of the aortic annulus. When a bioprosthetic valve is used, we believe that it is best to secure it to the Dacron graft 1 cm from one of its ends, as illustrated in Fig 7. The Dacron graft is then sutured to the aortic annulus with a continuous polypropylene suture, leaving a couple of millimeters of graft in between the sewing ring of the bioprosthetic valve and the aortic annulus. This technique permits future replacement of the bioprosthetic valve without taking down the coronary arteries from the Dacron graft.

When aortic valve homografts are used in patients with the Marfan syndrome, the aortic annulus often requires a reduction annuloplasty to match the size of the homograft available with the diameter of the aortic annulus. This can be done by plication of the sub-commissural triangles along the fibrous portion of the left ven-tricular outflow tract or by placing a band of Dacron graft on the outside of the aortic root along its fibrous portion, as illustrated in

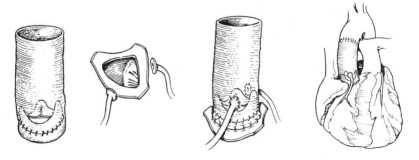

FIGURE 7.
Aortic root replacement with a stented bioprosthesis. The bioprosthetic valve is sutured 1 cm from the end of the graft. (From David TE: Surgery of the aortic valve. *Curr Probl Surg* 36:421-504, 1999. Used with permission.)

Fig 2. The homograft should be implanted in its anatomical position (ie, its muscular portion should correspond to the muscular portion of the recipient). The homograft can be safely sutured to the left ventricular outflow tract and aortic annulus with a continuous suture of polypropylene. The coronary arteries are reimplanted in their respective sinuses.

SURGICAL TREATMENT OF MITRAL REGURGITATION

Patients with the Marfan syndrome should have mitral valve surgery at the time of aortic root surgery if they have moderate or severe mitral regurgitation. Mitral valve surgery is sometimes performed in isolation in women with the Marfan syndrome and a normal aortic root. In patients with aortic root aneurysm and mitral regurgitation, the decision to replace 1 valve should not prevent repair of the other. Mitral valve repair is feasible in most patients with the Marfan syndrome.[3]

CLINICAL OUTCOMES

AORTIC VALVE–SPARING OPERATIONS

We recently published a comparison of outcomes of aortic valve–sparing operations with replacement of the aortic root in 78 patients with the Marfan syndrome.[7] There were 42 aortic valve–sparing operations and 36 aortic root replacements with mechanical and biological valves. There was only 1 operative death—that of a patient who had been in shock preoperatively because of end-stage aortic insufficiency with a massive ascending aorta that had aortic root replacement. The 10-year survival was 100% for the first group and 88% for the second (P = .04). Although this difference may be explained on the basis that patients who had aortic root replacement had higher functional class, larger aneurysms, more severe aortic insufficiency, and worse left ventricular function than did patients who had aortic valve–sparing operations, the data reinforces the view that patients with the Marfan syndrome should undergo earlier operation before developing aortic insufficiency and left ventricular dysfunction to optimize clinical outcomes. There were no reoperations on the aortic valve in the group who had aortic valve–sparing, and the freedom from reoperation in the aortic root replacement group was 64% at 10 years (P = .04). Reoperations were the result of infective endocarditis twice in 1 patient and biological valve failure in 3 patients.

Birks et al[10] reported on their experience with 82 patients with the Marfan syndrome who had aortic valve–sparing operations.

The 10-year survival was 84% for all patients; it was 64% for those with acute dissection and 75% for those with chronic dissection. The freedom from reoperation at 10 years was 83%. All patients in that series had remodeling of the aortic root without aortic annuloplasty. Because dilation of the aortic annulus is a progressive disease in patients with the Marfan syndrome, we believe this may be the cause of their relatively high reoperation rate.

MITRAL VALVE REPAIR
There are a limited number of reports on mitral valve repair in patients with the Marfan syndrome. We have performed it in only 23 patients from 1990 to 1999. There was no operative or late death. There have been no late failures, but the mean follow-up is only 39 months.

Fuzzelier et al[3] from the Broussais Hospital in Paris reported the results in 33 patients operated on from 1986 to 1996. There were 2 operative and 3 late deaths. At 10 years the survival was 79% and the freedom from reoperation on the mitral valve was 87%.

AORTIC ROOT REPLACEMENT
Gott et al[5] recently published the long-term results at 10 experienced centers of aortic root replacement in 675 patients with the Marfan syndrome. The 30-day mortality rate was 1.5% among the 455 patients who had elective surgery, 2.6% among 117 who had urgent surgery, and 11.7% among 103 who had emergency surgery. The survival rate was 75% at 10 years and 59% at 20 years. Dissection or rupture of the residual aorta and dysrhythmias were the leading causes of late deaths. Valve-related complications were as follows: The freedom from thromboembolic complications was 94% at 10 years, and the freedom from endocarditis was 95% at 10 years.

REFERENCES
1. Shores J, Berger KR, Murphy EA, Pyeritz RE: Progression of aortic dilatation and the benefit of long-term beta-adrenergic blockage in Marfan's syndrome. *N Engl J Med* 330:1384-1385, 1994.
2. Rossiter JP, Morales AJ, Repke JT, et al: A prospective longitudinal evaluation of pregnancy in the Marfan syndrome. *Am J Obstet Gynecol* 173:1599-1604, 1995.
3. Fuzzelier JF, Chauvaud SM, Fornes P, et al: Surgical management of mitral regurgitation associated with Marfan's syndrome. *Ann Thorac Surg* 66:68-72, 1998.
4. David TE, Omran A, Armstrong S, Sun Z, Ivanov J: Long-term results of mitral valve repair for myxomatous disease with and without

chordal replacement with expanded polytetrafluoroethylene sutures. *J Thorac Cardiovasc Surg* 115:1279-1286, 1998.

5. Gott VL, Greene PS, Alejo DE, et al: Replacement of the aortic root in patients with Marfan's syndrome. *N Engl J Med* 340:1307-1313, 1999.

6. Baumgartner WA, Cameron DE, Redmond JM, Greene PS, Gott VL: Operative management of Marfan syndrome: the Johns Hopkins experience. *Ann Thorac Surg* 67:1859-1860,1999.

7. Tambeur L, David TE, Unger M, Armstrong S, Ivanov J, Webb G: Results of surgery for aortic root aneurysm in patients with the Marfan syndrome. *Eur J Cardiothorac Surg* 17:415-419, 2000.

8. David TE, Armstrong S, Ivanov J, Omran A, Feindel CM, Webb G: Long-term results of aortic valve-sparing operations. *J Thorac Cardiovasc Surg*. In press 2000.

9. Furukawa K, Ohteki H, Cao JL, et al: Does dilatation of the sinotubular junction cause aortic insufficiency? *Ann Thorac Surg* 68:949-953, 1999.

10. Birks EM, Webb C, Child A, Radley-Smith R, Yacoub MH: Early and long-term results of a valve-sparing operation for Marfan syndrome. *Circulation* 100(suppl II):II29-II35, 1999.

11. Harringer W, Pethig K, Hagl C, Meyer GP, Haverich A: Ascending aortic replacement with aortic valve reimplantation. *Circulation* 100(suppl II):1124-1128,1999.

12. David TE: Aortic valve repair for management of aortic insufficiency. *Adv Cardiac Surg* 11:129-159, 1999.

13. David TE: Remodeling the aortic root and preservation of the native aortic valve. *Op Tech Cardiac Thorac Surg* 1:44-56, 1996.

14. David TE: Surgery of the aortic valve. *Curr Probl Surg* 36:421-504, 1999.

15. David TE, Armstrong S, Ivanov J, Barnard S: Surgery for acute type A aortic dissection. *Ann Thorac Surg* 67:1999-2001, 1999.

C HAPTER 4

Videoscopic Mitral Valve Repair and Replacement Using the Port-Access Technique

Eugene A. Grossi, MD
Associate Professor of Surgery, Division of Cardiothoracic Surgery, Department of Surgery, New York University School of Medicine, New York, NY

Angelo La Pietra, MD
Research Fellow in Cardiothoracic Surgery, Division of Cardiothoracic Surgery, Department of Surgery, New York University School of Medicine, New York, NY

Aubrey C. Galloway, MD
Professor of Surgery, Division of Cardiothoracic Surgery, Department of Surgery, New York University School of Medicine, New York, NY

Stephen B. Colvin, MD
Associate Professor of Clinical Surgery, Division of Cardiothoracic Surgery, Department of Surgery, New York University School of Medicine, New York, NY

The last 5 years have been an exciting and innovative time in the field of minimally invasive valvular heart surgery. The availability of endovascular technology to provide cardiopulmonary support, aortic cross-clamping, and cardioplegia delivery has freed surgeons from the necessity of having different cannulas entering through the thoracic incision.[1] As surgeons have made the transition away from the traditional sternotomy incision for mitral valve surgery, the comfort zone of the surgeon has moved from the large, omni-capable access of the midline sternotomy incision, to that of small thoracotomy with limited direct access.[2] Recently, the facilitating technology of endoscopy has been applied in the cardiac operating room to further enable this transition. The endoscope was recently reintroduced into the cardiac operating arena as a teaching device, such that the residents, medical students, and nurses in the operating room could view the operative target and observe what was transpiring during the procedure. As our familiarity with this technology has increased, surgeons are now making the transition from looking directly at the operative field to working from the view of the endoscopic monitor. This phenomenon has been described by Chitwood.[3] The final step in this transition is the current application of robotic instrumentation for mitral valve surgery. We are currently beginning to use robotic telemanipulators in the operating room to perform the procedure with the surgeon's total view being that of the robot's endoscopic video monitor. This chapter describes our current approach for minimally invasive mitral valve surgery and explains how endoscopic visualization has been integrated into our clinical practice.

VIDEO MONITORING FOR CARDIAC SURGERY

With the complexity of a cardiac procedure and the multiple video information sources in the operating room (vital-sign waveform monitors, overhead television cameras, headlight television cameras, echocardiographic imagery, endoscopic camera), it would be impossible and impractical to have a monitor dedicated to each of these video sources. Instead, we have several banks of monitors positioned both inside and outside of the operating room. Typically, there are 2 banks that consist of 2 monitors each, 1 bank on each of the lateral side walls of the operating room. This configuration of monitors allows the anesthesiologists, perfusionists, nursing staff, house staff, and the surgeon to have visual access to a bank of monitors from wherever they are standing, without the necessity for turning one's head. Additionally, there is a second bank of monitors outside of the operating room where students and visiting surgeons can easily observe and discuss the procedure without disrupting the surgical staff. The key to having this system work is a dedicated video matrix switch. This commercially available switch takes the various video inputs from the different sources and, depending on which part of the operation is taking place, displays the "active" images to the monitor banks. This video switch is typically controlled by the circulating nurse in the operating room. Additionally, one or more of the video sources can have input into a recorder for later review and editing.

PATIENT PREPARATION

Before preparing and draping the patient, the anesthesiologist places a transesophageal echocardiographic probe and, using this for guidance, introduces a percutaneous transjugular coronary sinus cardioplegic catheter. This is placed by an introducer in the right neck internal jugular vein. This technique is successful in greater than 85% of the cases. Positioning is done solely with transesophageal echocardiography.[4] When the catheter is in place and inflation of the balloon demonstrates ventricularization of the catheter's pressure wave form, a cine-fluoroscope is then momentarily brought into the operating room. A fluoroscopic picture (Fig 1) is taken to demonstrate that the catheter has not been advanced too far into the coronary sinus. During this initial preparation of the patient, one of the video monitors displays images from the overhead television camera, and the second monitor is used to display the transesophageal echo images.

One of the facilitators of doing videoscopic mitral valve surgery is the availability of a robotic voice-controlled endoscope. Although it is possible to have an assistant hold the endoscope or to attach it to an autoretraction device, the availability of the voice-controlled endoscopic robot (AESOP; Computer Motion, Santa Barbara, Calif) has greatly enhanced the experience. The single robotic arm, which clamps to the operative bed, can be positioned unobtrusively and will not interfere with the surgeons' approach to the mitral valve

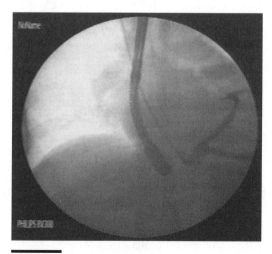

FIGURE 1.
Fluoroscopic picture to verify position of coronary sinus catheter to be used for retrograde cardioplegia.

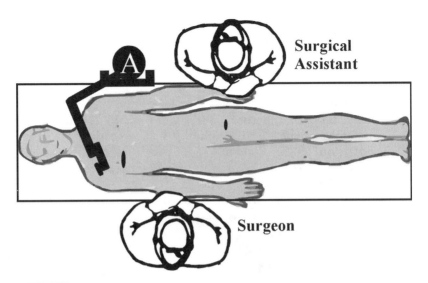

FIGURE 2.
Overhead view of operating room table demonstrating patient positioning and AESOP attachment.

(Fig 2). The patient is positioned in standard fashion, in the standard supine position on the operating table. The patient's right arm is draped over the head carefully so that the arm is protected, padded, and not under tension.[5] The patient is then prepared and sterilely draped. The robotic arm is also covered with a sterile sleeve at this time and incorporated into the sterile field.

OPERATIVE INCISIONS

After preparing and draping the patient, a small incision is made in the groin just above the skin crease to expose the femoral vessels. Because the patient has typically undergone cardiac catheterization in the right groin, we use the contralateral side (left). However, in smaller patients, sometimes there can be more difficulty with a left venous system approach. In advancing the venous cannula from the left groin, there is a sharper angle to traverse than on the right, as the left iliac vein has to cross the midline to the inferior vena cava. With the femoral vessels exposed through a 3-cm incision, attention is now turned to the chest. An inframammary skin incision is made on the right anterior chest, the lateral aspect of the incision starting at the anterior axillary line. It is approximately 3 fingerbreaths in length and is made directly over the fourth interspace in men. In women, the skin incision is made just underneath the skinfold of the breast, again with the lateral aspect of the incision starting at the anterior axillary line. The soft tissue is then retracted superiorly and a fourth intercostal incision is made. The intercostal muscles are divided both anteriorly and laterally to allow gentle opening of the interspace without the risk of fracturing the rib. Care is taken when advancing the intercostal incision medially so as to not injure the mammary veins or arteries. This incision provides direct exposure of the lateral wall of the pericardium. The diaphragm occasionally rides quite high with the patient in the supine position and may block the view of the inferior portion of the pericardium. This is dealt with by placing a zero silk suture through the tender portion of the diaphragm and passing it with the aid of a crochet hook through an angiocath placed in the seventh or eighth intercostal space. The tail ends of the silk suture are then pulled in an inferior position and snapped to the drapes with a clamp. This allows the diaphragm to retract inferiorly and helps to shift the lateral mediastinal contents into full view.

Into this incision, a soft-tissue retractor is placed (Heartport, Redwood City, Calif); this may seem unnecessary, but it is useful in keeping fatty debris from entering the operative field, as instruments tend to lie in contact with the walls of the incision. Subsequently, a small Finechetto retractor is placed to help expand the incision while avoiding unnecessary trauma to the ribs. A direct lateral incision is then made in the pericardium just about 1.5 cm anterior to the phrenic nerve. This is extended superiorly to the superior vena cava and inferiorly to the level of the diaphragm. With the pericardium opened, good visualization of the lateral wall of the right atrial appendage, the lateral wall of the right atrium, and the pulmonary veins is achieved.

CARDIOPULMONARY BYPASS

The patient is now fully heparinized and a small transverse incision is made in the femoral artery after clamping it proximally and distally with vascular clamps. By means of the Seldinger technique, an introducer and a guidewire are advanced into the femoral vessels, and the "endoreturn" catheter (Heartport) is advanced over the wire with no resistance. A snare is placed around the vessel, and a snared tourniquet is used to hold the vessel to the cannula. The arterial cannula is now connected to the arterial return from the pump, and the side arm of the cannula is cleared of air. Next, a clamp is placed across the cannula, and an endoclamp (previously prepared with a guidewire) is introduced into the opened valve of the side arm. The crossclamp is removed, and the occlusive fitting is snugged around the endoclamp, which is then

advanced to the 10 cm mark. The guidewire is advanced retrograde from the femoral artery into the descending aorta; the anesthesiologist turns the transesophageal echocardiogram probe to
monitor the descending aorta. The shepard's crook of the guidewire should easily be seen as it ascends the descending aorta (Fig 3).
As the top of the descending aorta is reached by the guidewire, the
echo is turned 180° to view the ascending aorta. Once the visualization of the guidewire in the ascending aorta is confirmed, the
end of the guidewire is held in a fixed position and the endoclamp
is threaded over it. Typically, the guidewire will advance into the
aortic valve somewhat and needs to be pulled back while under
constant surveillance. As the tip of the endoclamp reaches the
ascending aorta, its distinct profile is easily noted (Fig 4).

With all the cannulas in position, the patient is now placed on
full cardiopulmonary bypass. Typically, there are bilateral radial
arterial lines to measure the blood pressure. A balloon migration
would cause a differential in perfusion between the brachiocephalic and the left subclavian artery and would be detected by
a pressure differential between the radial lines. The pump flow

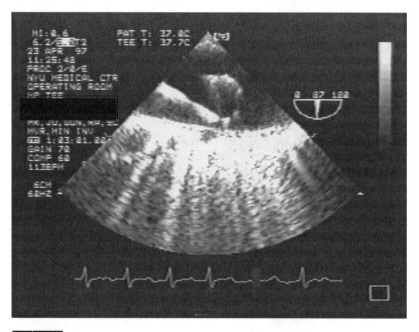

FIGURE 3.
Echocardiographic view of the guidewire in the descending aorta.

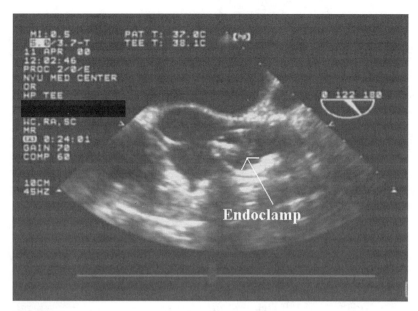

FIGURE 4.
Echocardiographic view of partially inflated endoclamp positioned in the ascending aorta.

rate is diminished to less than a liter per minute and the endoclamp balloon is inflated. This is done with visualization, under transesopageal echocardiographic guidance. The balloon, once inflated, is then snugged back slightly, being maintained in the ascending aorta while the main pump flow rate is turned up. This will help take any slack out of the endoclamp and position it securely in the aortic root just above a sinotubular ridge. During this procedure, once the balloon has been secured, retrograde cardioplegia is administered via the coronary sinus cardioplegic catheter. This gives excellent myocardial protection during the case. The aortic root is vented through the endoclamp.[1]

Through the small anterior thoracotomy, an incision is now made just anterior to the right pulmonary veins entering the left atrium. A cardiotomy pump sucker is placed here to evacuate the blood. This incision is extended superiorly and inferiorly. An intra-atrial retractor blade is now chosen to elevate the atrial septum. With the proper width and depth blade having been chosen, the handle for it is placed via a separate stab incision through the anterior chest, and the handle is now screwed into the blade and held in place by a self-retaining retractor. This provides excellent positioning of the atrial blade without using and tiring an assistant. Additionally, it keeps the retractor in a single place. Overzealous retraction by an assistant has the possibility of kinking the venous cannula as it travels through the right atrium and obstructing drainage from the superior part of the body. For this reason, vena cava pressures are monitored via the introducer side-port during the case. The intrathoracic field is flooded with carbon dioxide to reduce nitrogen entrapment inside the opened heart.

Attention is now turned to placing the endoscope in the operative field. A zero-degree 10-mm endoscope is our current preference. Because of temperature differentials inside the chest, it is advantageous to prepare the tip with a "no-fog" solution. In the same intercostal interspace incision but more posteriorly, a 10-mm trochar is placed through a stab incision in the skin. As mentioned previously, the intercostal incision has been extended posteriorly so as to facilitate atraumatic spreading of the ribs. This intercostal incision now is used for placement of the trochar. Under direct vision, the endoscope is advanced into the chest. The lateral cut edge of the left atrial tissue can sometimes present an obstacle. The endoscope should be advanced over the edge of the tissue and into the atrium. Typically, the tip of the endoscope is positioned within a distance of 6 to 7 cm from the plane of the mitral annulus. With the initial positioning of the endoscope performed manually, the AESOP robotic arm is swung over the table and attached to the endoscope holder. The surgeon can now concentrate on his operation. By speaking to the voice-controlled robotic arm, the surgeon can direct the endoscope to the appropriate area of the mitral annulus and leaflet currently being worked upon.

The surgeon, at this point, has the opportunity to work on the mitral valve either through his direct tunnel view (through the small anterior thoracotomy) or through the view provided on the endoscopic camera monitor (Fig 5). Because knots in this procedure typically are tied extracorporeally and slid into place using a knot-pusher (Heartport), the surgeon quickly finds that the videoscopic view provides excellent visual confirmation that the knots are coming together in an appropriate fashion. During this part of the procedure, a separate pump sucker is left in the pulmonary vein to evacuate any blood that may accumulate. The final reconstruction of the mitral valve can be visualized and tested with excellent exposure. There is no part of the mitral valve or annulus that cannot be precisely inspected (Fig 6). With the mitral reconstruction or replacement having been completed, the endoscope is withdrawn from the field and the trochar is removed. Now, 2 running

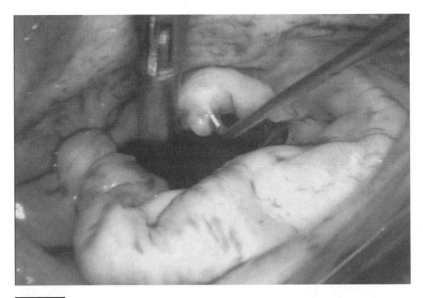

FIGURE 5.
Endoscopic view of the mitral valve. Severely prolapsing posterior leaflet is in forefield. Lengths of anterior leaflet chordae are being evaluated. Note anterior jet lesion (roughened endocardium) at base of anterior mitral leaflet.

sutures of nonabsorbable monofilament are used to close the atriotomy. Before doing this, a transvalvular vent is placed across the reconstructed or replaced valve into the left ventricle and placed on gentle suction. Next, a fibrillator cable is placed on the heart. The endoclamp balloon is slightly deflated enough to equalize the pressure in the ascending aortic root with the rest of the aorta. The central lumen of the endoclamp catheter is placed on suction, as is the left ventricular vent catheter. Gradient is placed in the heart while the heart is fibrillating. The lungs are manually inflated to help clear any potential air from the ventricle. The endoclamp is now fully reinflated, the electrical defibrillator disk is connected, and the heart is cardioverted. The heart is then allowed to beat against the occluding endoclamp while the ventricular vent is maintained on suction to clear any residual microbubbles in the blood from the ventricle. This continues under transesophageal echocardiographic guidance until it is visually demonstrated that all microcavitation has left the left atrium and the left ventricle. At this point, the endoclamp is fully deflated, and with the pump flow rate temporarily turned down, the endoclamp is removed.

The patient is now warmed to more than 35°C and weaned from the cardiopulmonary bypass machine. Before weaning from bypass, an epicardial ventricular pacing wire should be placed. From the small anterior approach, this can be exceedingly difficult to do once the heart is full of blood, and most typically should be done while the heart is still flaccid and under cardioplegic arrest.

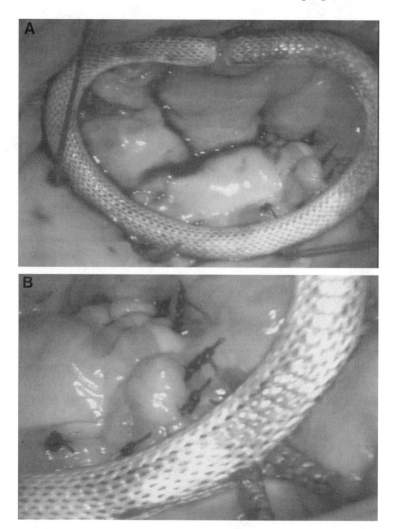

FIGURE 6.
A, Endoscopic view of completed mitral valve ring reconstruction. **B,** Magnified endoscopic view of the folding-plasty sutures of a mitral valve reconstruction.

Arterial decannulation follows the removal of the venous cannula and the administration of protamine. The femoral vessels are primarily repaired, and the thoracotomy incision is closed with a thoracostomy tube placed. Patients are not extubated in the operating room but brought to the recovery room where the muscle relaxants are reversed, and they are subsequently extubated within 1 to 2 hours.

RESULTS AND APPLICABILITY

This minimally invasive approach has had a major impact on the clinical approach to our patients. From January 1996 through March 2000, we have performed more than 1000 open heart procedures with the use of this minimally invasive technique. Mitral valves were reconstructed in 331 patients (68%) and replaced in 156 (32%). Previous cardiac surgery had been performed in 18.5% of these patients. Analysis of the first 100 isolated mitral valve reconstructions revealed no hospital mortality. During this initial experience, 13% of the isolated mitral patients did not have a minimally invasive approach, because they had severe atheromatous disease of the descending aorta and transverse arch. Subsequently, the availability of the "endodirect" balloon cannula allows the minimally invasive approach to be performed in patients with atheromatous disease.[6] At the first year follow-up, patients who underwent minimally invasive mitral reconstruction had equivalent echocardiographic results and improved clinical status as compared with the previous 100 patients at our institution who had mitral repair with the sternotomy approach.

Patient satisfaction with this approach is gratifying. We studied 25 patients with previous sternotomy and subsequent minimally invasive valve operation. These patients reported a 35% overall decrease in postoperative discomfort, a decrease in recovery time, and improvement in postoperative functional class with this minimally invasive approach. A subsequent prospective study revealed improved pulmonary function, decreased stress catecholamine levels, and improved postoperative function (Duke Activity Index) associated with the minimally invasive approach.[7]

During the past year, the videoscopic approach has been used extensively to enhance the surgical view of the mitral valve. We believe that while *not necessary* for minimally invasive mitral valve surgery, it enhances the procedure on several levels. The surgeon is provided with a detailed view of the structures being operated on. The residents, students, and operating room team can view the operation as it is being performed and can, therefore, participate as active assistants in the procedure. Alternatively, this video-scopic mitral approach is a very effective teaching tool, not only for the house staff to be able to review the procedures but also for visiting surgeons and satellite teleconferencing. Finally, this approach to the mitral valve is a necessary step as we begin to use robotic telemanipulators as part of the developing technology for minimally invasive mitral valve surgery.

REFERENCES

1. Schwartz DS, Ribakove GH, Grossi EA, et al: Minimally invasive mitral valve replacement: Port-access technique, feasibility, and myocardial functional preservation. *J Thorac Cardiovasc Surg* 113:1022-1031, 1997.
2. Colvin SB, Galloway AC, Ribakove G, et al: Port-access mitral valve surgery: Summary of results. *J Card Surg* 13:286-289, 1998.
3. Chitwood WR Jr: Video-assisted and robotic mitral valve surgery: Toward an endoscopic surgery. *Semin Thorac Cardiovasc Surg* 11:194-205, 1999.
4. Applebaum RM, Cutler WM, Bhardwaj N, et al: Utility of trans-esophageal echocardiography during port-access minimally invasive cardiac surgery. *Am J Cardiol* 82:183-188, 1998.
5. Falk V, Walther T, Autschbach R, et al: Robot-assisted minimally inva-sive solo mitral valve operation. *J Thorac Cardiovasc Surg* 115:470-471, 1998.
6. Glower DD, Komtebedde J, Clements FM, et al: Direct aortic cannula-tion for port-access mitral or coronary artery bypass grafting. *Ann Thorac Surg* 68:1878-1880, 1999.
7. Grossi EA, Zakow PK, Ribakove G, et al: Comparison of post-opera-tive pain, stress response, and quality of life in port access vs. stan-dard sternotomy coronary bypass patients. *Eur J Cardiothorac Surg* 16:39S-42S, 1999.

CHAPTER 5

Single-Stage Complete Unifocalization and Repair for Tetralogy of Fallot, Pulmonary Atresia, and Major Aortopulmonary Collateral Arteries

Kotturathu Mammen Cherian, MS, FRACS
Emeritus Professor in Cardiothoracic and Vascular Surgery, Tamil Nadu Dr. MGR. Medical University; Director, Institute of Cardiovascular Diseases, Madras Medical Mission, Chennai, India

Kona Samba Murthy, MCh
Senior Consultant, Institute of Cardiovascular Diseases, Madras Medical Mission, Chennai, India

Tetralogy of Fallot comprises 3.9% of congenital heart defects,[1] of which approximately 5% to 10% will have pulmonary atresia with ventricular septal defect (VSD). Two thirds of the cases with pulmonary atresia are associated with major aortopulmonary collateral arteries (MAPCAs).[2] Survival rate without surgery can be as low as 50% at 1 year of age and 8% at 10 years.[3]

Patients are initially seen with either cyanosis, caused by insufficient pulmonary blood flow, or congestive heart failure and pulmonary hypertension, caused by excessive pulmonary flow. A few patients may have a balanced pulmonary blood flow that permits them to survive to adulthood. Variation of pulmonary blood supply is the most distinctive feature in this anomaly. This is because the lungs develop from the foregut and their nutrient supply, as that of the esophagus, arises initially from the dorsal aortic plexus.[4] However, at about day 27 in the antenatal period, arterial branches of the paired 6th aortic arch form an anastomosis with the pulmonary vascular plexus. As a result, the lung receives dual supply. With time, the branches from the 6th arch enlarge, and those from the descending aorta become comparatively smaller. Persistence of the branches from the aorta in postnatal life forms the MAPCAs. They are variable in their origin, number, size, course, and arborization. The natural history of the MAPCAs often follows a course of progressive stenosis and occlusion. Thus, the sooner these collateral arteries are unifocalized and establish normal physiologic circulation, the greater number of healthier lung segments can be incorporated into the pulmonary circulation. The native pulmonary arteries (PAs) may be present or absent. If they are present, they are either normal sized or hypoplastic, or confluent or nonconfluent. An area of the lung may receive its blood supply from the native PA or MAPCAs either singly or in combination.

This complex subset of tetralogy remains one of the most challenging malformations to manage surgically. In an earlier period, these patients were treated with multistage unifocalization of MAPCAs through thoracotomies, followed by final repair via median sternotomy.[5-7] An aggressive approach involving single-stage complete unifocalization and complete repair through median sternotomy has been described by Reddy et al[8] and by us.[9] The surgical treatment for this malformation is evolving, and no standard protocols have been described. In this chapter, we describe in detail our surgical experience with single-stage complete unifocalization and repair, and discuss controversies associated with this new technique.

DIAGNOSIS

The initial diagnosis is made by means of echocardiography and confirmed with the use of cardiac catheterization and angiocardiography. An effort is made to obtain pressure measurements in individual MAPCAs. Selective angiographic delineation of MAPCAs is obtained in the ascending aorta, arch, descending aorta, and brachiocephalic arteries on either side. It is important to delineate the origin of each MAPCA and its course preoperatively in order to isolate each and plan the surgical options.

CLINICAL SPECTRUM

From June 1997 to April 2000, 40 patients were treated with single-stage complete unifocalization with or without final repair. Their ages ranged from 6 months to 23 years (median, 3 years), and weights ranged from 4 to 50 kg (median, 12 kg).

MORPHOLOGY

We identified 3 groups according to the morphological features of the PAs and MAPCAs and their arborization pattern in the lungs. Group I had well-formed PAs with MAPCAs, group II had hypoplastic PAs with MAPCAs, and group III had only MAPCAs without native PAs. The 3 groups were further subcategorized into those patients with protected MAPCAs with proximal stenosis, and those with unprotected MAPCAs (unobstructed flow)[10] (Figs 1-3). A total of 126 MAPCAs were unifocalized. The details of origin of the MAPCAs are shown in Table 1.

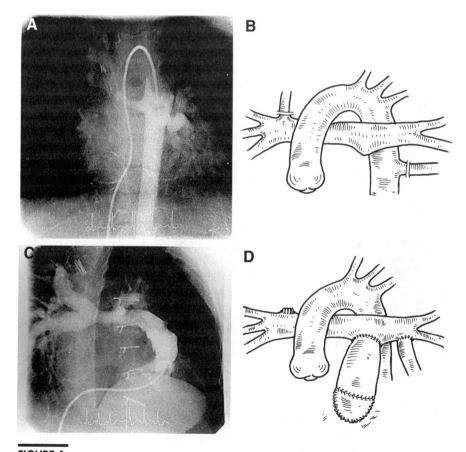

FIGURE 1.
Well-formed PAs with MAPCAs (group I). **A,** Preoperative angiography. **B,** Preoperative diagram. **C,** Postoperative angiography. **D,** Postoperative diagram. *Abbreviations: PAs,* Pulmonary arteries; *MAPCAs,* major aortopulmonary collateral arteries.

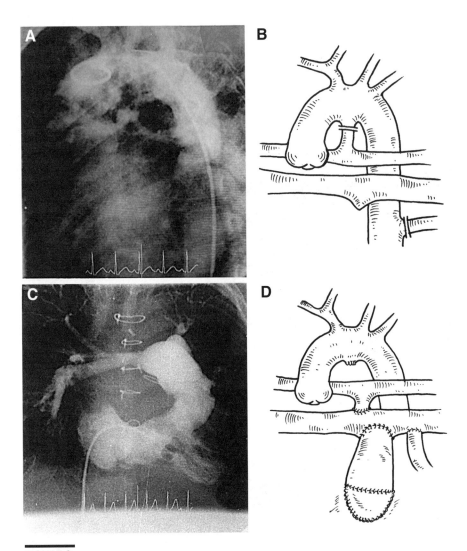

FIGURE 2.
Hypoplastic PAs and MAPCAs (group II). **A,** Preoperative angiography. **B,** Preoperative diagram. **C,** Postoperative angiography. **D,** Postoperative diagram. *Abbreviations: PAs,* Pulmonary arteries; *MAPCAs,* major aortopulmonary collateral arteries.

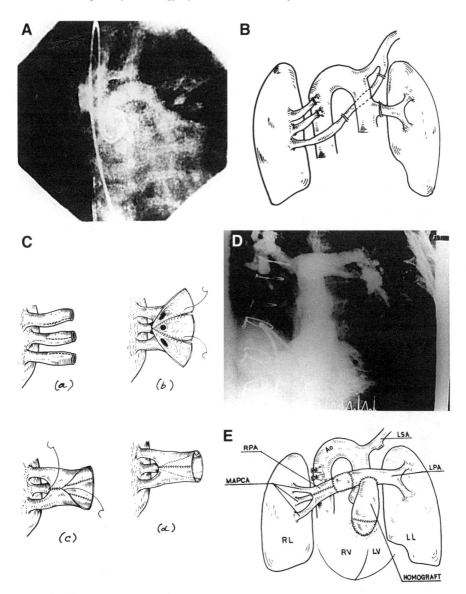

FIGURE 3.
Only MAPCAs (no native PAs, group III). **A,** Preoperative angiography. **B,** Preoperative diagram. **C,** Reconstruction of neopulmonary arteries. **D,** Postoperative angiography. **E,** Postoperative diagram. *Abbreviation: MAPCAs,* Major aortopulmonary collateal arteries. (Courtesy of Murthy KS, Shiva KN, Robert C, et al: Median sternotomy single stage complete unifocalisation for pulmonary atresia, major aortopulmonary collateral arteries and VSD: Early experience. *Eur J Cardiothorac Surg* 16:21-25. Copyright 1999, with permission from Elsevier Science.)

TABLE 1.

Profile of MAPCAs (n = 126)

Site of Origin	Occurrence
Descending aorta	76 (60.3%)
Arch	20 (15.9%)
Subclavian artery	28 (22.2%)
Ascending aorta	2 (0.6%)

Abbreviation: MAPCAs, Major aortopulmonary collateral arteries.

GOALS OF OPERATIVE THERAPY

Our aim was to establish a single source of blood supply to the lungs from PAs and MAPCAs, achieve tissue-to-tissue anastomosis, and avoid or minimize the use of prosthetic material in order to promote future growth in the children. Even though there might be dual supply in the lung if the MAPCAs were more than 2 mm in size, they were still unifocalized in order to maximize the pulmonary arterial bed available for final correction, on the assumption that the postoperative right ventricular (RV) pressure would be lower.[10]

TYPE OF SURGICAL PROCEDURE

All patients had single-stage complete unifocalization. According to availability of size and number of pulmonary vascular segments, they had one of the following 3 options of surgical treatment: (1) final repair (closure of VSD and RV-to-PA conduit), (2) RV-to-PA conduit alone (VSD left open), or (3) central shunt from ascending aorta to the reconstructed new PA with a polytetrafluoroethylene (PTFE) graft. If the size of the PA and MAPCAs was more than 75% of expected or more than 15 segments of the lung, final repair was done. If the size of the PA and MAPCAs was between 50% and 75% of normal or the pulmonary segments were between 10 and 14, an RV-to-PA conduit was employed without closure of the VSD. If the size was less than 50% of expected or PA segments were less than 10, only a central shunt was performed.[10]

INDICATIONS FOR OPERATION

The surgical management of this complex anomaly should be individualized according to (1) arborization of pulmonary vasculature, (2) amount of pulmonary blood flow, (3) morphology and sizes of the native PAs and MAPCAs, and (4) the age of the patient. The younger the age, the better the prognosis. In the protected PAs/MAPCAs (proximal stenosis), final repair or an RV-to-PA conduit or a central shunt should be done according to total availability and size of PAs. In hypoplastic or absent PAs with unprotected MAPCAs less than 1 year before they develop irreversible pulmonary vascular disease or protected MAPCAs with proximal stenosis, any one of the 3 surgical options is done according to the total size of the reconstructed new PAs. In patients with hypoplastic or absent PAs with unprotected MAPCAs, who are older than 1 year, all surgical options are questionable.[10]

SURGICAL TECHNIQUES
Median Sternotomy

After routine median sternotomy, pericardium was harvested for subsequent use. The native PAs (if present) were dissected and isolated to their hilar region. The ascending aorta and the superior vena cava (SVC) were freed from surrounding tissues in order to retract them freely to get satisfactory access to the deeper plane for dissection. The MAPCAs were approached by dissecting along the aorta and the brachiocephalic arteries, as per their course delineated by preoperative angiography, to a sufficient length from their origin to bring them to the transverse sinus without any tension during anastomosis. Opening of the pleura was not necessary because of limited dissection. The descending aortic MAPCAs were reached by dissecting in the posterior mediastinum after opening the posterior pericardium. In the left arch, the descending aortic MAPCAs were approached by dissecting between the area of the left side of the ascending aorta and left atrium, and above or below the left main bronchus (Fig 4). While dissecting on the left side, care was taken not to compress the left coronary artery and its branches during retraction. In the right arch, the descending aortic MAPCAs were reached by approaching between the ascending aorta, SVC, and the roof of the left atrium, usually above or below the carina and right main bronchus (Fig 5). During the dissection, care was taken to avoid hemodynamic compromise by momentarily stopping the dissection and retraction. Precautions were taken not to injure the trachea, bronchi, esophagus, and phrenic, vagus, and recurrent laryngeal nerves (Fig 6). All the MAPCAs were looped before initiating cardiopulmonary bypass (CPB).

Under CPB and beating heart, all the MAPCAs were disconnected from their origin and the proximal ends were closed. They were anastomosed end to side or side to side to native PAs if present; otherwise, MAPCAs to MAPCAs (Figs 1-3). Anastomosis was

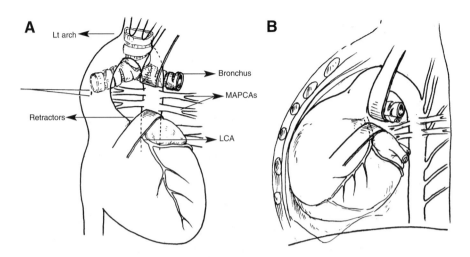

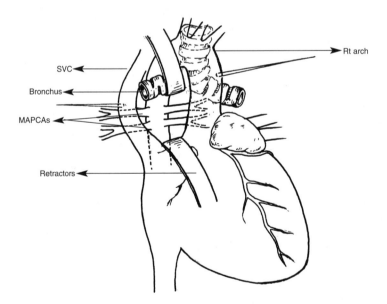

FIGURE 4.
Dissection of descending thoracic aortic MAPCAs in left aortic arch. **A,** Anterior view. **B,** Lateral view. *Abbreviations: MAPCAs,* Major aortopulmonary collateral arteries; *Lt,* left; *LCA,* left coronary artery.

FIGURE 5.
Dissection of descending thoracic aortic MAPCAs in right aortic arch. *Abbreviations: SVC,* Superior vena cava; *MAPCAs,* major aortopulmonary collateral arteries; *Rt,* right.

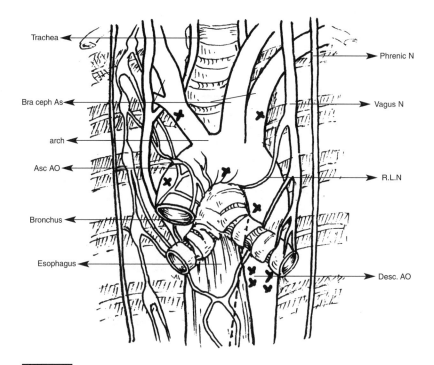

FIGURE 6.
Important mediastinal structures (*X mark* showing the site of origin of MAPCAs). *Abbreviations:* MAPCAs, Major aortopulmonary collateral arteries; *N,* nerve; *RLN,* recurrent laryngeal nerve; *Asc Ao,* ascending aorta; *Desc Ao,* descending aorta; *Bra ceph As,* brachiocephalic arteries.

done by using 8-0 polypropylene continuous sutures. Tissue-to-tissue anastomosis was preferred to allow future growth in the children. Under cardioplegic arrest, the VSD was closed with a PTFE patch, and RV-to-PA continuity was established with a cryopreserved aortic or pulmonary homograft conduit. If the resultant MAPCA-PA diameter was not suitable for complete repair, the VSD was left alone or a central shunt was done from the ascending aorta to the PA with a PTFE interposition graft on a beating heart.

Clamshell Approach

In the clamshell approach, through a submammary skin incision, extending laterally to the anterior axillary line, both the pleural cavities were entered through the fourth intercostal space. The internal mammary artery and vein were ligated and divided on either side. The sternum was divided transversely. The remainder

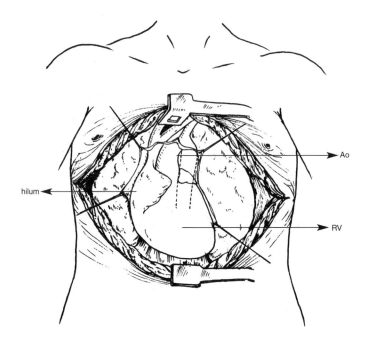

FIGURE 7.
Clamshell approach. *Abbreviations: Ao,* Aorta; *RV,* right ventricle.

of the dissection and subsequent procedure was similar to that of the median sternotomy approach. This technique was used for patients who had undergone a previous surgical intervention, such as median sternotomy for a central shunt or an attempted surgical repair. Previous surgical intervention results in extensive scarring of the tissue around the mediastinum and the hilar region. In the clamshell approach, there is no need for extensive dissection. It gives excellent exposure to both hilar regions, the heart, and the great vessels (Fig 7).

RESULTS
EARLY RESULTS

A median sternotomy was used for 36 patients, and a clamshell approach was used for 4 patients. All patients had single-stage complete unifocalization. The postoperative results are shown in Table 2.

Forty patients had 45 procedures (1.1 procedures/patient). All patients had single-stage complete unifocalization, of whom 58% had final repair (VSD closure and RV-to-PA conduit), 25% had an RV-to-PA conduit alone (VSD left open), and 17% had a central shunt. Tissue-to-tissue anastomosis was achieved in all patients except one, in whom a 14-mm PTFE tube graft was used to achieve the confluence of the PAs. The mean CPB time was 148 ± 29 minutes (range, 114–208), and the mean aortic cross clamp time was 45 ± 21 minutes (range, 15-95). In the final repair group, the mean ratio of RV to left ventricular (LV) pressure (PRV/LV ratio) was 0.66 (range, 0.38–0.9), and the systemic oxygen saturation ranged from 95% to 100%. In patients in whom the VSD was left open and an RV-to-PA conduit or a central shunt was done, the systemic saturation ranged from 85% to 96% (mean, 92%) and 72% to 88% (mean, 78%), respectively.

MORTALITY AND MORBIDITY

There were 6 early deaths (15%). There were no deaths in group I and 3 deaths each in groups II and III. The first patient had complete unifocalization and final repair and could not come off bypass because he had suprasystemic RV pressure. He was placed back on bypass and the VSD patch was removed. He had prolonged bypass time, developed RV dysfunction, and died on the seventh postoperative day. The second death was of a 1-year-old child who had complex unifocalization and an RV-to-PA conduit without VSD closure. His saturation was maintained between 85% and 92% with an F$_{IO_2}$ (fraction of inspired oxygen) of 0.3. A low cardiac output gradually developed, and he died on the second postoperative day. At autopsy a 4-mm MAPCA in the lower part of the descending aorta was noted, which was missed on preopera-

TABLE 2.
Results

Group	Complete Unifocalization	Final Correction	RV-to-PA Conduit	Central Shunt	Mortality
Total N = 40	All	23 (58%)	10 (25%)	7 (17%)	6 (15%)
Group I N = 14	All	14 (all)	—	—	Nil
Group II N = 12	All	4	5	3	3
Group III N = 14	All	5	5	4	3

Abbreviations: RV, Right ventricle; *PA,* pulmonary artery.

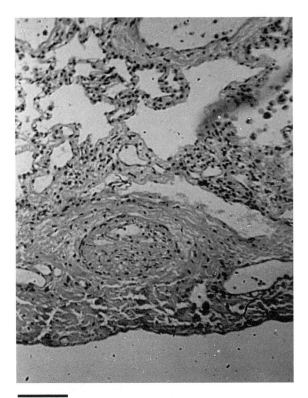

FIGURE 8.
Grade III (Heath Edwards) pulmonary vascular changes.

tive angiography. The third patient was a 7-year-old boy with unprotected MAPCAs without native PAs who had complete unifocalization and an RV-to-PA conduit. Gradual desaturation and ventricular failure developed, and he died on the fourth postoperative day. At autopsy the lung specimen showed grade III pulmonary vascular changes according to the Heath Edwards classification (Fig 8). The fourth patient died of intractable bleeding on the first postoperative day. Another 2 patients died of low cardiac output and multiorgan failure. Four patients had reexploration for excessive mediastinal bleeding. Two patients had unilateral phrenic palsy, and 1 patient had bilateral phrenic palsy and required prolonged ventilation.

FOLLOW-UP

The follow-up ranged from 1 to 35 months. All patients had echocardiography to assess RV function, conduit position, and distal PA diameter at the time of discharge, and regular follow-up (Figs 1-3).

The first 16 patients had cardiac catheterization and angiocardiography either before they were discharged from the hospital or after 3 months of the first follow-up to assess the status of the repair. The patients who had an RV-to-PA conduit without VSD closure had cardiac catheterization and angiocardiography performed within 3 to 12 months of the initial operation. Indications for completion of VSD closure were congestive heart failure requiring decongestive therapy, improved resting oxygen saturation by pulse oximeter, and a predominant left-to-right shunt demonstrated by echocardiography. These findings were confirmed by cardiac catheterization. If the left-to-right shunt was greater than 2:1, with an increased shunt fraction on 100% FIO_2, the VSD was closed.

There were 5 reoperations. Four patients had successful completion of VSD closures, and 1 patient had reconstruction of pulmonary stenosis (a PTFE graft was used to achieve the pulmonary confluence). There were 3 late deaths. Two of these patients developed a progressive increase in RV pressure and died 2 and 2½ years, respectively, after the initial operation. Endocarditis developed in one patient, who died 2 months after surgery.

DISCUSSION

Patients with tetralogy of Fallot, pulmonary atresia, and MAPCAs remain one of the most challenging groups to manage surgically. Untreated, most patients will die early in life, either with severe cyanosis and its attendant complications or with congestive heart failure and progressive pulmonary vascular disease. In an earlier period, these patients were treated with conventional multistage procedures. Previously published data show that multistage procedures require an average of 3 procedures (range, 2-6) before complete repair. This culminated in final repair in 11.5% to 60.5% of patients. Overall mortality while achieving complete repair has ranged from 10.2% to 19.2%.[5-7] From 1993 to May 1997, these patients were treated with multistage unifocalization in our institute. Fourteen patients had 21 procedures (1.5 procedures/patient), in which only 3 of them had complete repair. There were 2 deaths (14%).[9]

The microvasculature of the lungs in patients with MAPCAs is healthier at birth. The natural history of MAPCAs often follows a course of progressive stenosis and occlusion, sometimes precluding access to a given segment of the lung. Long-standing severe stenosis may lead to distal arterial hypoplasia and underdevelopment of preacinar and acinar vessels and alveoli.[11] In staged unifocalization, the use of nonviable conduits with a tendency to occlusion may lead to a loss of lung segments. Infancy is characterized by the highest rate of attrition, and without surgery, almost 50% of patients die before 1 year of age. Any surgical procedure designed to have an impact on the natural history of these patients must alter the pattern of attrition in infancy. If delayed staged unifocalization is done, only 20% to 30% of a cohort of newborns will achieve final repair. Most staged approaches are based on the concept of an initial phase to increase the native PA blood flow in an effort to stimulate growth. Various strategies have served to advance the field and have provided some good results in a select group of patients, but many patients remain without final repair. When the staged approach is used, it is difficult to achieve final repair in patients with nonconfluent hypoplastic and absent native PAs.[6]

For that reason, an aggressive approach consisting of single-stage unifocalization and repair has been started.[8,9] From June 1997 onward, we began performing single-stage unifocalization. Forty patients have been treated with this technique. There was no mortality among patients in group I (those with well-formed PAs and MAPCAs). There were 3 deaths each in groups II and III, indicating that these 2 groups are the difficult spectrum regarding decision making, surgical technique, and development of progressive disease.

Fifty-eight percent of the total group had final repair, 25% of the patients had an RV-to-PA conduit, and 17% of the patients had a central shunt. Four patients had completion of VSD closure. In the McElhinney group,[12] 64% of the patients had final repair. Their ages ranged from 2 weeks to 37 years (mean, 7.3 months), and 65% were younger than 1 year. In that experience, the follow-up ranged from 1 to 61 months. There were 6 late deaths, and 14 patients underwent completion of VSD closure. In our experience, the follow-up ranged from 1 to 35 months. There were 3 late deaths and 4 patients underwent completion of VSD closure as a final repair. In both experiences, the primary aim is to achieve tissue-to-tissue anastomosis for future growth. Both the groups use calcium-supplemented warm blood prime to maintain the beating heart during the unifocalization procedure.

There were some differences between our approach and that of the Hanley group. We used a routine median sternotomy incision in usual cases and the clamshell approach in previous sternotomy patients for unifocalization. We dissect the MAPCAs from their origin to a sufficient length to reach for the anastomosis. The dissection is limited, and injury to the phrenic nerve and other important structures may be less. Opening of the pleura is rarely necessary to identify the MAPCAs for dissection.[10] In Hanley's technique, a generous midline median sternotomy incision is used. Both the pleural spaces are opened widely anterior to the phrenic nerves and the lungs are lifted out of the pleural cavities, allowing identification of the collaterals at their aortic origins.[8] We choose the type of surgery, such as final repair, an RV-to-PA homograft, or a central shunt, according to the total size of the PAs and MAPCAs and their segmental distribution as shown by angiocardiography and intraoperative assessment. In Hanley's technique, intraoperative pump flow is used to check the PA pressure and accordingly decide the type of surgery. If arborization is inadequate, it would be better not to close the VSD. Even though there is a correlation between the total neopulmonary artery index (TNPAI; Nakata index[13]) and the postoperative PRV/LV ratio, there was a substantial overlap in the TNPAI below 200 mm^2/m^2.[17] It is difficult to estimate the Nakata index because of arborizational abnormalities, technical problems in reconstruction of neopulmonary arteries, and distal MAPCA stenosis.

CONTROVERSIES

Patients with unobstructed MAPCAs have the same clinical course as do other patients with aortopulmonary shunts, such as those who have truncus arteriosus or aortopulmonary window. In patients with unobstructed MAPCAs, we suggest surgical intervention before the age of 1 year, before irreversible pulmonary vascular changes or MAPCA stenosis develop.[10,13] Two patients in our experience died with suprasystemic RV pressures at 2 and 2½ years after final repair. They had a progressive increase in RV pressure even though the immediate postoperative PRV/LV ratio was 0.7. and 0.4, respectively. We presume that these patients had progressive pulmonary vascular disease. Based on that experience, we began fenestrating the VSD patches in final repair patients.

In our experience, the patients who had a central shunt (pulmonary vascular segments < 10) have not shown much improvement in pulmonary vascular growth and did not come for final repair or at least for RV-to-PA conduit (Fig 9). It is doubtful whether surgical intervention in these patients changes the natural history of TOF, pulmonary atresia and MAPCAs. It is difficult to repair all multiple distal stenoses of the MAPCAs (Fig 10). Other extreme forms occur in which there are no demonstrable native PAs or MAPCAs by angiocardiography. Instead, multiple small

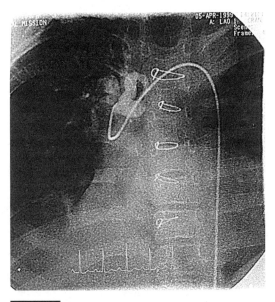

FIGURE 9.
Angiography of unifocalization and central shunt.

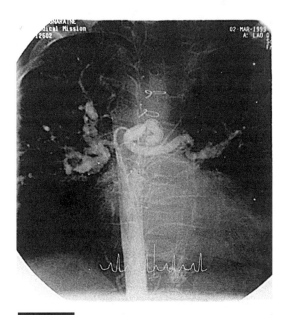

FIGURE 10.
Angiography of MAPCAs with multiple distal stenoses. *Abbreviation: MAPCAs,* Major aortopulmonary collateral arteries.

collaterals are present that supply both the lungs. These patients present with severe cyanosis. We feel that in these patients also, we are not able to offer any surgical intervention to improve their condition.

CONCLUSION

With single-stage unifocalization, patients are able to undergo complete repair, preferably at an early age. Complete repair achieves early normalization of cardiovascular physiology with correction of cyanosis or pulmonary hypertension and attendant complications. Early single-stage unifocalization reduces the number of operations and hospitalizations, and thereby is less expensive than a multi-stage procedure. By achieving tissue-to-tissue anastomosis, we can expect future growth in these children. Approaching the MAPCAs through a median sternotomy or a clamshell incision is safe and reproducible. Early and midterm results are encouraging, and ongoing follow-up will allow identification of those patients who will benefit from surgery.

REFERENCES

1. Kenna AP, Smithells R, Hielding DW: 1975 congenital heart diseases in Liverpool. *Q J Med* 43:2-44, 1960-69.
2. Shimazaki T, Maec hra T, Blackstone EH, et al: The structure of the pulmonary circulation in tetralogy of Fallot with pulmonary atresia. *J Thorac Cardiovasc Surg* 95:1048-1058, 1988.
3. Bertnou EG, Blackstone EH, Hazelerig JB, et al: Life expectancy without surgery in tetralogy of Fallot. *Am J Cardiol* 42:458–466, 1978.
4. Huntington GS: The morphology of pulmonary artery in the mammalia. *Anat Rec* 17:165-201, 1919.
5. Puga FJ, Leoni FE, Julsrud PR, et al: Complete repair of pulmonary atresia, ventricular septal defect and severe peripheral arborization abnormalities of central pulmonary arteries. *J Thorac Cardiovasc Surg* 98:1018-1029, 1989.
6. Iyer KS, Mee RB: Staged repair of pulmonary atresia with ventricular septal defect and major systemic to pulmonary artery collaterals. *Ann Thorac Surg* 51:65-72, 1991.
7. Marelli JA, Perloff KJ, Child SJ, et al: Pulmonary atresia with ventricular septal defect in adults. *Circulation* 89:243-251, 1994.
8. Reddy VM, Liddicoat RJ, Hanley LF: Midline one stage completes unifocalization and repair of pulmonary atresia with ventricular septal defect and major aorto pulmonary collaterals. *J Thorac Cardiovasc Surg* 109:832-845, 1995.
9. Murthy KS, Rao SG, Shivaprakasha KN, et al: Evolving surgical management for VSD, pulmonary atresia and major aorto pulmonary collateral arteries. *Ann Thorac Surg* 67:760-764, 1999.

10. Murthy KS, Shiva KN, Robert C, et al: Median sternotomy single stage complete unifocalisation for pulmonary atresia, major aorto pulmonary collateral arteries and VSD: Early experience. *Eur J Cardiothorac Surg* 16:21-25, 1999.
11. Rabinovitch M, Herrera, De Leon, et al: Growth and development of the pulmonary vascular bed in patients with tetralogy of Fallot with or without pulmonary atresia. *Circulation* 64:1234–1249, 1981.
12. McElhinney DB, Reddy VM, Hanley FL: Tetralogy of Fallot with major aorto pulmonary collaterals. Early total repair. *Pediatr Cardiol* 19:289-296, 1998.
13. Nakata S, Imai Y, Takanashi Y, et al: A new method for quantitative standardization of cross sectional areas of the pulmonary arteries in congenital heart diseases with decreased pulmonary blood flow. *J Thorac Cardiovasc Surg* 88:610-615, 1984.
14. Reddy VM, Petrossian E, McElhinney DB, et al: One stage complete unifocalization in infants: When should the ventricular septal defect be closed? *J Thorac Cardiovasc Surg* 113:858-868, 1997.

CHAPTER 6

Gene Therapy for Coronary Artery Disease

Todd K. Rosengart, MD

Associate Professor of Surgery, Northwestern University Medical School;
Head, Division of Cardiothoracic Surgery, Evanston Northwestern
Healthcare, Evanston Hospital, Evanston, Ill

Katherine Hillebrand

Research Assistant, Northwestern University Medical School, Evanston
Hospital, Evanston, Ill

A growing body of evidence continues to lend support to the application of biological revascularization strategies to treat coronary atherosclerotic disease.[1] As such, the treatment of adult heart disease soon may be entering a period of major change. Currently, myocardial ischemia and its sequelae are treated with antianginal medications, to reduce myocardial oxygen demand; with medications and lifestyle measures, to prevent further disease progression; with angioplasty and stent placement (percutaneous coronary interventions), thrombolysis, and coronary artery bypass grafting (CABG), to restore blood flow to a segment of the epicardial coronary artery; and, more recently, with transmyocardial laser revascularization (TMLR), to channel oxygenated blood to ischemic regions.

Despite the relative effectiveness of these therapies, coronary artery disease (CAD) remains the leading cause of mortality and morbidity in the Western world.[2,3] Angioplasty and surgical bypass are the primary interventions for atherosclerosis, but these therapies are limited by the development over time of native-vessel restenoses and graft occlusions.[4] Coronary-artery restenosis occurs in 10% to 30% of initially successful percutaneous coronary interventions, and CABG is associated with recurrent disease in about 50% of cases at 10 years.[5] Traditional therapies also are not options for the significant number of patients who have especially diffuse and widespread vascular pathology, who have poor targets for grafts, or who have chronic total occlusion. Multiple restenosis, degenerated saphenous-vein grafts, absent conduits after bypass surgery, small distal vessels, severe calcification of the aorta, or severe chronic obstructive pulmonary disease are other potential contraindications.[2,4] For these patients, inducing the heart to reperfuse itself may be the best option. Angiogenesis, the growth of new vasculature, is a critical biological response to ischemia that provides collateralization, or "biological revascularization" around vascular obstructions.[4] Site-specific gene transfer can be used to modulate vascular disorders in a physiologically meaningful way, including therapeutic angiogenesis.[1,3,4,6]

ANGIOGENESIS

The growth of new blood vessels is a native process, occurring naturally as part of wound healing; tissue remodeling, repair or regeneration; corpus luteum formation; the normal endometrial cycle; and in response to ischemia. Angiogenesis is the predominant mechanism for increasing collateral blood flow in chronic myocardial ischemia.[7] Various mediators induce angiogenesis, such as growth factors known as "angiogens." Therapeutic angiogenesis is a strategy of administration of one or more exogenous angiogens to tissues where angiogenesis is desired, to augment native angiogenic processes and enhance formation of collateral vasculature.[4]

Angiogenesis involves the sprouting or splitting (intussusception) of capillaries and small nonmuscular vessels from existing capillaries.[7,8] Although debate persists as to the exact mechanisms underlying new blood-vessel growth and development, one schema suggests that capillary collaterals develop by sprouting (angiogenesis), whereas muscular collaterals develop in situ from existing arterioles (arteriogenesis).[9] In contrast, vasculogenesis refers to the *de novo* embryological development of blood vessels from angioblasts and mesodermal precursors.[7,8] The observation that reduction of angiogen expression is lethal in embryonic life highlights the critical role played by angiogens.[8]

In postnatal development, collateralization forms "autobypass" conduits, bridging from the stem arteries to re-entrant vessels downstream. This process occurs, for example, in patients with atherosclerotic obstructions. Collateral-vessel formation improves regional perfusion and function of the ischemic myocardium. Epicardial collaterals may help maintain perfusion by enlargement of existing arterioles.[7] In contrast, subendocardial perfusion may be restored by true angiogenesis as opposed to the recruitment of native vessels.[7] Enhanced angiogenesis may help improve angina and myocardial function in patients with advanced coronary atherosclerosis and myocardial ischemia, improve wound healing, and prevent tissue loss in patients with peripheral ischemia.[1]

In normal adult coronary arteries, endothelial and vascular smooth-muscle cells are mitotically inactive.[7] During growth and development and during ischemia, hypoxia, inflammation, or other stresses, these cells begin to migrate and divide.[7] The capillary endothelial cell is the only cell type that can express all the necessary information for the formation of new microvascular networks; it achieves this in concert with monocytes, smooth-muscle cells, mast cells, lymphocytes, pericytes, neutrophils, and fibroblasts.[4] During this process, the endothelial cells revert to a proliferative phenotype but later return to the quiescent phenotype. Control of this process appears to relate to the differential expression of various angiogenic agonists and antagonists.

During angiogenesis, endothelial cells replicate, form network capillaries, and connect with the existing vasculature. The steps in this complex process, only partially understood, are as follows: The intracellular and extracellular signaling pathways are activated. The release of cell-derived proteolytic enzymes and increased vascular permeability initiate angiogenesis by lysing the adhesion molecule "glue" between the endothelial cells and the underlying basement membrane of the parent vessel. Degradation is induced by proteases such as collagenase and plasminogen activators. Once the bond between the endothelium and surrounding extracellular matrix is degraded, the endothelial cells freely migrate, proliferate, and remodel. The endothelial cells are guided by chemotactic properties along an angiogen concentration gradient. By adhesion and reattachment, the endothelial cells form a lumen, generating sprouts from the parent vessel. These organized, 3-dimensional, tube-like structures elongate from the tip to form capillaries. Pericytes migrate along the newly formed endothelial cell lumen. The new capillaries network with the existing arterial and venous systems to re-establish cell-cell interactions and form solid connections to re-establish flow. The endothelial cells then revert to the nascent vascular phenotype. The endothelial cells, having formed a primitive vascular bed, are surrounded by smooth-muscle cells to complete the growth of the vessel.[3,4,7,10,11]

HOMEOSTASIS OF ANGIOGENESIS

Angiogenesis is a critical component for fetal development, but the activity of angiogenic growth factors must be modulated by inhibitory proteins after birth. Neoplasms, for example, appear to require growth-factor expression to maintain tumor growth. Under normal conditions, angiogenesis is highly regulated and occurs only with imbalances between the supply and demand of oxygen and nutrients to a vascular bed or with inflammation.[7] As such, angiogenesis can be induced by traumas such as ischemia, hypoxia, cell injury, and cell death, but after a period of days to weeks, it is down-regulated once an appropriate angiogenic response has begun.[4] An interface between normal and ischemic or hypoxic tissues may contribute or be critical to the angiogenic process. As part of this process, inflammation itself appears to lead to new blood-vessel growth, especially during infection and neoplasia.[7]

Although angiogenesis can occur as a natural response to ischemia or stress, it typically cannot completely prevent ischemia or infarction from acute vascular occlusions.[12] Reasons for this include insufficient local generation of cytokines and reduced responsiveness of atherosclerotic endothelium to growth factors.[10] For this reason, gene therapy and other strategies may be of critical benefit in expediting and aiding angiogenesis in the diseased myocardium and other tissues.

MODULATORS OF ANGIOGENESIS

The cornerstone of all angiogenic therapies is the observation that the simple addition of an angiogenic substance (angiogen) can stimulate the cascade of events inducing angiogenesis.[4] Of the many substances now known to induce angiogenesis, the two most-investigated are within the vascular endothelial growth factor (VEGF) and fibroblast growth factor (FGF) families of polypeptide growth factors.

ANGIOGENIC GROWTH FACTORS

The VEGFs are a family of potent angiogens first isolated as a heparin-binding factor secreted from bovine pituitary folliculostellate cells.[6] Also known as vascular permeability factor because of its ability to induce capillary leakage and thereby produce tissue edema, VEGF is distinguished from other known angiogens by 2 features: (1) it is a mitogen almost exclusively for endothelial cells (as opposed to smooth-muscle cells and fibroblasts) and (2) it has, at its amino-terminus, a signal sequence that permits natural secretion by intact cells.[11] Its high-affinity binding sites, the receptors R-1 and R-2 (flt-1 and flk-1), are present almost exclusively on endothelial cells, making it specific for those cells. Relevant to the therapeutic application of VEGF, ischemia stimulates expression of both VEGF and its receptors. This could allow a targeted therapeutic response in ischemic tissues while reducing the potential for pathological angiogenesis elsewhere.[13]

There are 4 known isoforms of VEGF, containing 121, 165, 189 or 206 amino acids, of which VEGF-165 predominates.[13] Heparin-binding ability increases as the size of the isoform increases.[3,4] Although most studies have examined the 121 and 165 residue forms of VEGF (VEGF-A), other structural forms, such as VEGF-B, -C, -D, -E, and -F, also are being investigated.

Like VEGF, the prototypical fibroblast growth factors (aFGF and bFGF; acidic and basic, respectively) are heparin-binding polypeptides. These FGFs are single chains of 154 (aFGF) and 146 (bFGF) amino acids.[3] High-affinity FGF receptors activate intracellular signaling pathways responsible for initiation of cell replication.[4] The FGF receptors have widespread expression; thus, the FGFs are mitogenic for a variety of cell types: endothelial cells, smooth-muscle cells, fibroblasts, myocytes and certain tumor cells.[4] There is consequently a risk of fibrosis or intimal hyperplasia with these more widespread FGFs.

More than 20 other angiogenic proteins also have been identified,[3] including angiogenin, platelet-derived growth factor (PDGF), platelet-endothelial cell adhesion molecule (PECAM), hepatic/hepatocyte growth factor (HGF), scatter factor (SF), leptin, thrombopoietin/thrombospondin, proliferin, hypoxia-inducible factor 1 (HIF-1), transforming growth factors alpha and beta, tumor necrosis factor-alpha, interleukin-8 and possibly human growth hormone (hGH). Numerous other "cofactors" also appear to be critical in the normal process of angiogenesis.

HEPARIN

The ability of many growth factors to bind heparin likely prolongs their bioavailability for induction of angiogenesis. This property of the heparin-binding growth factors promotes binding to the cell surface, and matrix heparan sulfates create a biological reservoir of the secreted protein, enhancing the temporal opportunity for bioactivity.[11] In addition, heparin protects many growth factors from degradation. Although heparin itself is not an angiogen, it is an important angiogen cofactor, presumably due to these processes.[4]

ANGIOPOIETINS (ANG-1 AND ANG-2)

The angiopoietin-tie-2 receptor system also appears to play a critical role in angiogenesis and development of the cardiovascular system.[3] The two major ligands for the tie-2 receptor are angiopoietin-1 and -2 (ang-1 and ang-2). Acute administration of ang-1 prevents leakage from the adult vasculature, countering the potential permeability actions of VEGF and inflammatory agents.[14] Ang-1 does not appear to induce angiogenesis unless used in combination with VEGF, but ang-1 appears to be an important angiogenic cofactor, causing "maturation" and stabilization of the vasculature.[8]

Ang-2 is the naturally occurring antagonist of ang-1. Ang-2 likely plays an integral role early during blood-vessel formation. In human beings, it is expressed at locations of vascular remodeling; ang-2 has been found to be concentrated at the leading edge of growing vessels.[15] It has been suggested that angiogenesis is aided by inhibition of tie-2 by ang-2; the resulting vasculature becomes destabilized and thus is more responsive to angiogenic factors such as VEGF.[16]

NITRIC OXIDE (NO)

There is a strong relation between the release of nitric oxide and regulation of blood-vessel growth and development, although the exact roles of NO in the different stages of angiogenesis have not been determined and differ between species and vascular beds. VEGF is a potent stimulant for the release of nitric oxide, and VEGF's NO-induced vasodilation augments flow. NO induces angiogenesis in vivo, causes proliferation of postcapillary endothelial cells in tissue culture, and is involved in tube formation.[7]

Nitric oxide synthase (NOS), the enzyme responsible for endothelial NO production, also appears to be a potential angiogenic cofactor. Both VEGF and FGF have been shown to activate angiogenesis in the presence of NOS.[17] Studies on the therapeutic efficacy of NOS, however, have been contradictory thus far; some have shown that NOS overexpression can lead to neointimal formation of diseased or balloon-injured atherosclerotic arteries, whereas others have shown reduced mural inflammation and lipid accumulation in the presence of NOS.[17] In the presence of NOS inhibitors, the proliferative effect of VEGF is decreased, but other studies have shown increases in NOS inhibitors when angiogenesis was induced.[7]

DELIVERY OF ANGIOGENS TO TARGET TISSUES

Both protein- and gene-based therapies have been shown to enhance the angiogenic response to ischemia and tissue reperfusion. Whether it is more effective to deliver angiogens by direct protein administration or by a plasmid, adenovirus, or other viral vector is unknown.[1]

PROTEIN THERAPY

Direct administration of an angiogenic protein has the merit of simplicity, since it does not require incorporation of a gene into the nucleus, as is necessary in gene therapy.[7] Slow release of a recombinant protein, by using polymer, heparin-alginate, or other sustained-release formulations, may prolong high concentrations of growth factor without the potential risks associated with viral vectors.[8] Administration of the protein alone has the disadvantage of requiring relatively larger amounts of angiogen to be injected. Theoretically, administration of large doses of protein could allow leakage to other parts of the body and induce angiogenesis in unwanted tissues. Targeting the "take" of the protein also may be difficult.

GENE THERAPY

Gene therapy involves administration of complementary deoxyribonucleic acid (cDNA) "instructions" inserted into plasmids or viral vectors, to induce endogenous production of the protein of interest. Gene therapy encoding for the protein may be preferable over protein therapy for several reasons. Gene therapy spurs the body's own cells to produce growth factors in "microphysiological" quantities. In contrast, administration of pharmacological doses of angiogenic proteins may unbalance angiogenic processes.[18] Gene therapy theoretically allows expression of the angiogen of interest for longer intervals than does protein therapy. Thus, direct tissue administration of angiogenic proteins by gene therapy may both minimize systemic side effects, such as hypotension with VEGF and nephrotoxicity with bFGF, and provide slow release of the encoded factor. This could lead to an enhanced angiogenic response compared with the potentially short exposure to growth factor associated with protein-based therapy.[8]

Gene therapy is effected primarily through simple DNA moieties or viral vectors. Theoretical disadvantages relate to the low efficiency of DNA-based strategies and the host's immune response to viral vectors, both of which interfere with host-cell transfection. In contrast to proteins that remain intracellular (such as bFGF), however, genes that encode for secreted proteins (such as VEGF) potentially can overcome the handicap of inefficient transfection. This occurs through a paracrine effect and results in secretion of proteins sufficient to achieve biologically meaningful levels.[6,11] Viral vectors, although clearly more efficient than naked DNA, also remain limited by potential local and systemic toxicities.[17] When choosing the appropriate vector for gene therapy, it is important to determine how much angiogen is necessary and how long expression of the angiogen needs to continue for therapy to be effective.

As opposed to most current strategies, which employ in vivo gene therapy, ex vivo gene therapy describes a process whereby homologous cells are harvested, transfected with the angiogen cDNA in vitro, and readministered to targeted tissues.[4] Ex vivo therapy is limited by its cumbersome nature and the risk of introducing infection to the host organism and the heart. It is well suited, however, for use in cardiac transplantation and in saphenous-vein harvesting. The tissue to be implanted is perfused with the angiogen outside the body before implantation, which ensures transfection without the risks of systematic transgene administration.[3] The efficacy of ex vivo therapy for angiogenesis remains to be explored more fully.

PLASMIDS

Plasmids are cDNA linked covalently into a circular structure. Because the cDNA does not have to be encapsulated in a separate vehicle for entry into the cell, the size of the transgene is not limited. The plasmid DNA contains a promoter that "turns on" transcription of the plasmid transgene, such as the gene that codes for a growth factor. Means of delivering the plasmid include simple contact; physical means, such as pressurized delivery and pellet-penetration strategies ("gene guns," for example); or chemical means, such as lipophilic or hydrophobic compounds.[4] The use of plasmid DNA is inefficient, successfully transfecting less than 1% of targeted smooth-muscle cells,[11] but adjunctive measures can aid transfection. Despite low transfection efficiency, a gene that encodes for a secreted protein such as VEGF may be of therapeutic benefit. Ischemia and other stresses also may augment the transfection efficiency of cDNA.[6] The advantage of plasmid as opposed to viral gene therapy is that minimal immunity is built up to the plasmid vector, so readministration is not limited. Because the plasmid DNA is taken up by endosomes and then degraded by lysozymes when it enters the cell, only about 0.1% is transported to the cell nucleus.[3,4] The relatively large quantities of plasmid required to overcome the low transfection efficacy could increase the risk of plasmid "spillage" and remote promiscuous angiogenesis.

RETROVIRUSES

These ribonucleic acid (RNA) viruses are the largest gene therapy vectors and thus can accommodate large expression cassettes. Retroviruses contain a reverse transcriptase, which converts viral RNA into proviral DNA. The viral DNA is transported into the host-cell nucleus, where it randomly and permanently integrates into the genome and codes for lifelong expression (for the cell's lifetime). The potential advantage is prolonged expression, but there is a risk of mutagenesis as with any foreign DNA incorporation into the host genome. Retroviruses can be used only for replicating cells. This makes them relatively less useful for therapeutic angiogenesis, because most target cells are in a postreplicative state.[4] Lentiviral vectors have been created to infect nondividing cells, however, and may be applicable for cardiovascular diseases.[17]

REPLICATION-DEFICIENT ADENOVIRUS
The adenoviruses are composed of a double-stranded, linear DNA genome and core proteins surrounded by capsid proteins. A wild-type adenovirus typically is made incapable of replication by 1) deleting the E1 and E3 regions of the vector gene that control replication and 2) inserting the transgene of interest and any necessary promoters into that space. The virus inserts the selected transgene into myocytes, which then become "minifactories" producing, for example, the angiogenic growth factor. With direct tissue delivery, adenoviral-based gene therapy provides sustained, localized transgene expression. Immune responses, among other potential mechanisms, limit the persistence of the transgene over time. This limiting factor can be advantageous, however, because it prevents prolonged expression and minimizes the risk of unwanted or excessive angiogenesis.[4]

Several properties of adenoviruses make them potentially ideal for angiogenic therapy. Like plasmids, adenoviruses assume an epichromosomal location, which avoids the risk of permanent alteration of the cellular genotype or insertional mutagenesis.[3] The adenovirus vector also is more efficient than plasmids at transfecting target cells. Adenovirus can be applied to nonreplicating cells; retroviruses cannot. Prolonged VEGF in skeletal tissue has been shown to cause hemangiomas, so a shorter term of expression likely would be advantageous, and adenoviral-mediated expression lasts only for 1 to 2 weeks. Adenoviruses have a high affinity for receptor tissues, and purified preparations appear not to induce inflammation. Thus, they appear ideal for therapeutic applications.

ADENO-ASSOCIATED VIRUSES
The adeno-associated viruses (AAVs) are small members of the parvovirus family. They provide much longer transgene expression than adenoviruses, probably because they become efficiently integrated into the host genome or because the vector induces less immunity than do adenoviruses. AAV-derived vectors have the advan-

tages of being nonpathogenic and noninflammatory, allowing stable, long-term expression. The size of the AAV genome makes it difficult to insert genes that code some of the larger transgenes, however.

METHODS OF DELIVERY

Protein or gene therapy can be given by the perivascular, intravascular, intramuscular, or subcutaneous route. In localized therapy, the selected angiogen or vector is administered directly into tissues in immediate proximity to the area targeted for angiogenesis, usually by intramuscular or subcutaneous injection of the protein. Localized therapy theoretically reduces the risk of remote toxicity. Localized intravascular delivery by various catheter systems, however, holds the potential for systemic leakage.

In systemic therapy, the angiogen is given from a distance, by intravenous or intraarterial injection. Systemic therapy avoids the difficulty of accessibility with some target sites, such as the myocardium. There are risks associated with systemic delivery and with angiogen leakage into systemic circulation from the local delivery site. Systemic leaks could cause promiscuous angiogenesis in undesirable, remote sites, such as the retina and synovium, or promote the growth of occult tumors. Systemic administration also increases the risks of global hemodynamic derangements, increased vascular permeability, hypotension, and edema.[4] Systemic therapy is used because it is assumed that angiogenesis will occur only in wounded or ischemic areas where angiogenesis is desired. Wounded and ischemic tissues are poorly perfused and subject to reduced blood flow, however, so accessibility to these tissues is limited when using systemic-delivery strategies. Evidence also exists to support the likelihood of angiogenesis in nonischemic tissues.

CLINICAL TRIALS

Perhaps 10% to 20% of patients with symptomatic obstructive CAD and documented ischemia are not candidates for traditional methods of revascularization. An estimated 5% of patients would be eligible for newer methods of therapy, following the most rigorous inclusion criteria of the U.S. Food and Drug Administration-approved drug angiogenesis protocols: ejection fraction of at least 25%, documented ischemia in at least 20% of the left ventricle, and angina class 2 or greater.[2]

GENE THERAPY FOR CAD

Clinical trials of gene therapy for CAD have included adjunct-to-bypass and minimally invasive, "gene therapy alone" trials.

Common to all clinical trials of gene therapy for CAD are their promising initial results: decreases in angina class and nitroglycerin use, angiographic or other evidence of collateralization or enhanced perfusion, and the lack of systemic or local inflammatory reactions.

In a viral-based approach to angiogenic gene therapy, AdVEGF121 (adenovirus encoding the VEGF-121 isoform) has been used successfully in Phase I clinical safety trials and appears to be well tolerated in patients with clinically significant CAD.[19,20] We have observed no evidence of systemic or cardiac adverse advents related to vector administration for up to 6 months after adenovirus-based therapy. Furthermore, 30 days after vector administration, coronary angiography and stress sestamibi scanning suggested improved wall motion.[19]

In a plasmid-based gene-therapy strategy, patients with chronic severe angina underwent direct intramyocardial gene transfer of naked DNA coding for VEGF165 (phVEGF) as the sole therapy.[21,22] All patients had marked improvement in symptoms, showing decreases in anginal frequency and severity. Nitroglycerin use decreased in all patients, and 70% were completely free of angina at 6 months. All patients had objective evidence of improved myocardial perfusion and collateral flow, as demonstrated by coronary angiography and by nuclear perfusion scans with single-photon emission computed tomography (SPECT) at rest and during stress.[6,17]

CONCERNS ABOUT ANGIOGENESIS

Because angiogenesis is a developing field, many potential risk factors need further exploration. Pathological angiogenesis can cause proliferative retinopathies, rheumatoid arthritis, and tumor development, for example.[3] To date, however, no such peripheral side effects have been reported.[21-23]

Concern has arisen about the link between angiogenesis and malignancy, because as tumor cells grow, they may overexpress one or more of the positive regulators of angiogenesis. Tumor cells mobilize angiogenic proteins from the extracellular matrix, or they recruit host cells such as macrophages, which produce their own angiogenic proteins.[10] Tumor cells must recruit endothelial cells from the surrounding stroma to form their own endogenous blood supply, driven by the tumor's metabolic requirements.[3] Angiogenesis therefore could stimulate tumor growth because it increases the number of angiogenic factors available to the tumor. There is a theoretical possibility, but no cases thus far, of VEGF augmenting the growth of small dormant tumors or interfering with surveillance for malignant cells.[7]

In addition, there are concerns about whether plaque formation depends on angiogenesis. High concentrations of circulating angiogens could stimulate plaque angiogenesis and secondary plaque growth.[10] Expression of VEGF and its receptors has been correlated with severity of atherosclerosis in human coronary arteries, and local administration of FGF has led to unfavorable arterial remodeling in injured coronary arteries.[17,24] In this regard, adenoviral gene transfer was shown to induce thrombosis in atherosclerotic rabbit arteries, but not in normal arteries.[17,24] If angiogenesis is crucial to plaque formation, the identification of antiangiogenic factors might help eliminate the stenosis that is the basis of CAD.[25] This potential risk of angiogenic therapy, however, remains only theoretical at present.

Finally, VEGF, because it increases vascular permeability, can increase risks associated with vascular leakage. Pathological increases in vascular leakage can lead to edema and swelling, causing potentially serious problems in patients with brain tumors, diabetic retinopathy, stroke, sepsis, and inflammatory conditions such as rheumatoid arthritis and asthma.[14] Again, no such toxicity has yet been observed.

THE FUTURE OF GENE THERAPY FOR HEART DISEASE

The exact stimulus for angiogenesis remains controversial. Initial data, however, support the potential of angiogenic therapy for growth of new collateral vessels in the heart. This promising therapy may be able to reduce mortality and morbidity after coronary-artery occlusion.[7] Future applications of gene therapy in the heart may include adjunctive treatment for TMLR or CABG or as a sole treatment delivered by catheter.

Gene therapy has yet to overcome some potentially critical hurdles, such as vector-related inflammation, limited expression spans, suboptimal delivery systems, and varying gene-expression levels.[17] The best growth factor or combination, the correct dosage, the easiest means of delivery, the ideal route of administration, and the means to prevent toxicity all must be determined before gene therapy can enjoy widespread use. As an alternative to gene therapy, protein-based strategies are another option.[26]

It is unknown whether an angiogenic treatment will be sufficient for prolonged periods or whether periodic "boosters" will be necessary to maintain benefit. Repeated administrations during cardiac catheterization, invasive surgery, thoracoscopy, or minimally invasive techniques may be required. Alternatively, regulatable gene therapy with chronic expression vectors may prove useful.[27] Young and healthy animals have greater responses to protein or gene therapy than do older patients with atherosclerotic disease; challenges to bridging this gap remain. Therapeutic angiogenesis probably will not replace bypass surgery and angioplasty, but it likely will be available to augment these traditional interventions.

REFERENCES

1. Rosengart TK: New approaches to the surgical therapy of atherosclerotic coronary artery disease. *Am J Cardiol* 83:40B-45B, 1999.
2. Mukherjee D, Bhatt DL, Roe MT, et al: Direct myocardial revascularization and angiogenesis-how many patients might be eligible? *Am J Cardiol* 84:598-600, 1999.
3. Hamawy AH, Lee LY, Crystal RG, et al: Cardiac angiogenesis and gene therapy: a strategy for myocardial revascularization. *Curr Opin Cardiol* 14:515-522, 1999.
4. Rosengart TK, Patel SR, Crystal RG: Therapeutic angiogenesis: protein and gene therapy delivery strategies. *J Cardiovasc Risk* 6:29-40, 1999.
5. Bailey SR: Local drug delivery: current applications. *Progr Cardiovasc Dis* 40:183-204, 1997.
6. Losordo DW, Vale PR, Isner JM: Gene therapy for myocardial angiogenesis. *Am Heart J* 138:132-141, 1999.
7. Hariawala MD, Sellke FW: Angiogenesis and the heart: therapeutic implications. *J R Soc Med* 90:307-311, 1997.
8. Ferrara N, Alitalo K: Clinical applications of angiogenic growth factors and their inhibitors. *Nat Med* 5:1359-1364, 1999.
9. Iwakura A, Komeda M, Fujita M: Coronary stenosis and mechanisms of collateral vessel growth. *Japan J Clin Med* 56:2504-2508, 1998.
10. Gibaldi M: Regulating angiogenesis: a new therapeutic strategy. *J Clin Pharmacol* 38:898-903, 1998.
11. Isner JM: Angiogenesis for revascularization of ischaemic tissues. *Eur Heart J* 18:1-2, 1997.
12. Sellke FW, Simons M: Angiogenesis in cardiovascular disease: current status and therapeutic potential. *Drugs* 58:391-396, 1999.
13. Henry TD: Can we really grow new blood vessels? *Lancet* 351:1826-1827, 1998.
14. Thurston G, Rudge JS, Ioffe E, et al: Angiopoietin-1 protects the adult vasculature against plasma leakage. *Nat Med* 6: 460-463, 2000.
15. Maisonpierre PC, Suri C, Jones PF, et al: Angiopoietin-2, a natural antagonist for tie2 that disrupts in vivo angiogenesis. *Science* 277:55-60, 1997.
16. Peters KG: Vascular endothelial growth factor and the angiopoietins: working together to build a better blood vessel. *Circ Res* 83:342-343, 1998.
17. Sinnaeve P, Varenne O, Collen D, et al: Gene therapy in the cardiovascular system: an update. *Cardiovasc Res* 44:498-506, 1999.

18. Anonymous: Heart disease-therapy spurs growth of new blood vessels. *Harv Heart Lett* 23:4-5, 1998.
19. Rosengart TK, Lee LY, Patel SR, et al: Angiogenesis gene therapy: phase I assessment of direct intramyocardial administration of an adenovirus vector expressing VEGF121 cDNA to individuals with clinically significant severe coronary artery disease. *Circulation* 100:468-474, 1999.
20. Rosengart TK, Lee LY, Patel SR, et al: Six-month assessment of a phase I trial of angiogenic gene therapy for the treatment of coronary artery disease using direct intramyocardial administration of an adenovirus vector expressing the VEGF121 cDNA. *Ann Surg* 230:466-470, 1999.
21. Losordo DW, Vale PR, Symes JF, et al: Gene therapy for myocardial angiogenesis: initial clinical results with direct myocardial injection of phVEGF165 as sole therapy for myocardial ischemia. *Circulation* 98:2800-2804, 1998.
22. Symes JF, Losordo DW, Vale PR, et al: Gene therapy with vascular endothelial growth factor for inoperable coronary artery disease. *Ann Thorac Surg* 68:830-836, 1999.
23. Patel SR, Lee LY, Mack CA, et al: Safety of direct myocardial administration of an adenovirus vector encoding vascular endothelial growth factor 121. *Hum Gene Ther* 10:1331-1348, 1999.
24. Staab ME, Simari RD, Srivatsa SS, et al: Enhanced angiogenesis and unfavourable remodeling in injured porcine coronary artery lesions: effects of local basic fibroblast growth factor delivery. *Angiology* 48:753-760, 1997.
25. SoRelle R: Two sides of the same coin: Stop angiogenesis for cancer and encourage it for coronary artery disease. *Circulation* 98:383-384, 1998.
26. Hendel RC, Henry TD, Rocha-Singh K, et al: Effect of intracoronary recombinant human vascular endothelial growth factor on myocardial perfusion: Evidence for a dose-dependent effect. *Circulation* 101:118-121, 2000.
27. Prentice H, Bishopric NH, Hicks MN, et al: Regulated expression of a foreign gene targeted to the ischaemic myocardium. *Cardiovasc Res* 35:567-574, 1997.

CHAPTER 7

Optimal Temperature for Routine Cardiopulmonary Bypass*

Richard M. Engelman, MD
Professor of Surgery, University of Connecticut School of Medicine, Farmington, Conn; Clinical Professor of Cardiothoracic Surgery, Tufts University School of Medicine, Medford, Mass; and Chief, Cardiac Surgery, Baystate Medical Center, Springfield, Mass

Edward D. Verrier, MD
Chief, Division of Cardiothoracic Surgery, University of Washington Medical Center; William K. Edmark Professor of Cardiovascular Surgery, Vice Chairman, Department of Surgery, University of Washington School of Medicine, Seattle

With the development of normothermic myocardial preservation more than 10 years ago,[1] the advantage of hypothermic systemic perfusion for cardiopulmonary bypass (CPB) to assist in the maintenance of myocardial hypothermia became no longer a clinical imperative. In fact, the ability to safely conduct CPB at normothermia was now an issue to be addressed.

An excellent review of the influence of temperature on cerebral perfusion and metabolism during CPB documented how closely cerebral oxygen consumption is linked to perfusion temperature, decreasing approximately 7% for every 1°C reduction in temperature.[2] Cerebral perfusion during nonpulsatile bypass is determined mainly by the mean arterial pressure, a function of both the systemic flow rate and the vascular resistance. In fact, as temperature is reduced, increased systemic vascular resistance results in the redistribution of blood flow to the brain, maintaining adequate perfusion. It has been well known for some time that the effect of hypothermia is to afford significant cerebral protection

*Supported in part by the National Institutes of Health (grant RO1 HL-48631).

from ischemia during CPB.[3] This effect is manifested by both decreased high-energy phosphate degradation and inhibition of excitatory neurotransmitter release during induced ischemia.[4] However, a point of diminishing returns can occur such that mild hypothermia ($>28°C$) can allow cerebral blood flow (CBF) to remain in excess of metabolic demands,[5] whereas a more profound degree of systemic hypothermia ($<24°C$) may lead to impaired cerebral autoregulation and increased cerebral vascular resistance.[6]

Systemic hypothermia during CPB naturally requires rewarming, and there are a number of reports in the literature describing the dangers of systemic hyperthermia, even if only at the level of $39°C$.[7] In fact, rewarming hyperthermia is difficult to avoid, leading to cerebral oxygen deprivation and measurable jugular venous desaturation.[8] The risk of this scenario is the probable potentiation of the acceleration of an ischemic cerebral insult, which is clearly best to avoid. In essence, both systemic hypothermia ($<24°C$) and hyperthermia ($>38°C$) have deficiencies. A randomized prospective trial was thereby recently completed by our group at the Baystate Medical Center to answer neurologic issues regarding the optimal perfusate temperature for routine CPB.

HISTORICAL DEVELOPMENT

Successful CPB is dependent on a range of mechanical processes that provide the necessary substitution of an artificial method for oxygen delivery and carbon dioxide removal, and the need to pump blood sufficient to maintain the circulation. First and foremost is the absolute necessity to prevent blood from clotting while circulating outside the body and the requirement to return the circulation to its initial normally coagulant state. Jay McLean,[9] as a medical student at Johns Hopkins, first reported on the discovery of heparin, describing its anticoagulant properties in 1916. More than 20 years later, in 1937, Chargaff and Olson[10] discovered protamine, thus providing the means for accomplishing successful clinical perfusion by reversing the effects of heparin.

The development of blood pumps began in 1928 with a valved device delivering a pulsatile wave.[11] In 1934, the DeBakey[12] roller pump, now the standard on which all positive displacement pumps have been modeled, was described. The development of oxygenators for clinical extracorporeal perfusion has rapidly matured from rotating screen or disk oxygenators,[13] to bubble oxygenators,[14] to membrane oxygenators,[15] and most recently to the hollow fiber membrane,[16] which significantly reduces the total surface area required for gas exchange. These advances have come about in concert with improved blood pumps, particularly the centrifugal pump, which avoids the occlusive processes of the positive displacement pumps, inherently reducing blood trauma.[17]

Perfusion temperature in the early years of CPB has been an issue primarily related to providing adequate perfusion and oxygenation, particularly when oxygenation and carbon dioxide withdrawal have been less than adequate. Hypothermia reduces systemic metabolism, and any lack of adequate perfusion constitutes a reason to reduce perfusion temperature. When CPB was first developed, perfusion was not adequate for maintaining metabolic processes, which in and of itself was the principal reason to use hypothermic perfusion. However, because our present perfusion techniques are adequate for complete systemic metabolic support, this is no longer valid.

Perfusion temperature during bypass has also been an issue because normothermia requires relatively high flow rates in the range of 100 to 120 mL/kg per minute, equivalent to basal cardiac output.[18] This may be associated with troublesome coronary and pulmonary collaterals that hinder surgical exposure, lead to substantial cardiotomy suction, and prevent maintenance of induced arrest.[19] Ultimately, the use of lower flow rates, intentional hemodilution, and hypothermia became standards of practice.[20] In the 1970s, the techniques of myocardial preservation generally adapted myocardial hypothermia as an optimal approach based on the early work of Shumway et al[21] and the scientific support of Buckberg et al.[22] With the presumed need for myocardial hypothermia during preservation, there was an impetus to maintain systemic hypothermia to avoid collateral myocardial rewarming.

With the advent of warm preservation in 1990[23] and the use of blood cardioplegia, whether warm, tepid, or cold, the requirement of cold perfusion no longer existed. It is now accepted that optimal myocardial preservation does not require systemic hypothermia, and warm or tepid perfusion can be used safely. In addition, we now know that there is more than a 90% reduction in myocardial oxygen demand upon arrest of electromechanical activity with cardioplegia, even if the myocardium is only moderately hypothermic (-22°C).[22-24] It is therefore the influence of perfusion temperature on the physiologic processes that determines an optimal perfusion temperature for routine perfusion, with a major issue remaining as the uncertainty regarding the neurologic implications of perfusion temperature.

CEREBRAL METABOLISM

CPB has traditionally been performed with hypothermic perfusion because the decreased temperature results in lowered tissue metabolism, imparting both implied myocardial and cerebral protection.[25] In the brain, perfusion temperature directly relates to cerebral metabolism, with a reduction in cerebral oxygen consumption of approximately 7% for every 1°C reduction in temperature.[2] A recent study of the effects of normothermic (37°C) or hypothermic (27°C) perfusion on the brain was reported in which CBF and cerebral arteriovenous oxygen difference were specifically measured.[26] This allowed calculation of the cerebral metabolic rate for oxygen ($CMRO_2$, cerebral oxygen consumption), the cerebral oxygen delivery (CDO_2), and the CDO_2 to $CMRO_2$ ratio (the adequacy of oxygen delivery). Also measured was cerebral vascular resistance.

The major findings of this random study in 60 patients were:

1. Global cerebral oxygenation is well maintained under normothermic conditions. An increase in CBF maintains CDO_2 at the prebypass level despite hemodilution. There remains a close coupling of oxygen demand and delivery. This is not true during hypothermia.
2. During hypothermic bypass (27°C), the coupling of $CMRO_2$ and CBF or CDO_2 is not maintained. Whereas CDO_2 is decreased during hypothermia, $CMRO_2$ undergoes a greater decrease, and the ratio of CDO_2 to $CMRO_2$ increases significantly, indicating oxygen delivery in excess of demand.
3. After completion of bypass, both normothermic and hypothermic groups, now both rewarmed, demonstrate high CBF and low cerebral vascular resistance while $CMRO_2$ is at baseline in both groups. These postoperative changes are probably secondary to persistent hemodilution. After bypass in both warm and cold groups, cerebral oxygen supply and demand are well matched.

The results of this study support the safety of normothermic or warm perfusion. During warm bypass, there is persistent coupling of cerebral oxygen demand and delivery that is lacking in the hypothermic patient. It is not known at what perfusion temperature this appropriate coupling of cerebral oxygen demand/supply no longer applies, but it is anticipated that tepid perfusion at 32°C to 34°C maintains this coupling process. Moreover, with further reduction in perfusion temperature to 20°C to 24°C (true hypothermia), cerebral pressure–flow autoregulation is impaired and cerebral vascular resistance increases.[6] This may, in and of itself, potentially induce cerebral ischemia if perfusion pressure is even transiently decreased during bypass, which is a common occurrence during CPB.

NEUROLOGIC AND NEUROPSYCHOLOGICAL FUNCTION AFTER CPB

At the Baystate Medical Center, we recently reported on a clinical research study that had as its primary goal the correlation of perfusion temperature with neurologic function after CPB.[27] In this National Institutes of Health (NIH)-funded trial completed in 1998, 291 patients of 1777 screened were enrolled in a randomized trial of hypothermic (20°C), tepid (32°C), or warm (37°C) perfusion during routine CPB for patients requiring 3 or more coronary artery grafts. Each patient received a neurologic examination by a "blinded" dedicated neurologist using a test vehicle termed the modified Mathew Scale (Table 1), before operation, 4 days after operation, and at 1-month follow-up. This test examines 3 aspects of neurologic function, cognition, elemental skills, and disability. A total of 267 patients completed all 3 neurologic examinations.

Eligibility for the trial required that the patient be younger than 76 years and have no prior neurologic history. If a carotid bruit was

TABLE 1.
Mathew Scale for Neurologic Evaluation

Evaluation	Score
Cognitive function	
Consciousness	0-8
Orientation	0-6
	0-14
Elemental skills	
Language	0-23
Motor	0-20
Reflexes	0-3
Sensorium	0-3
Visual field	0-3
Gaze preference	0-3
Facial weakness	0-3
	0-58
Disability	
Functional capacity	0-28
Total	0-100

audible, the patient had a duplex scan, and any patient with a carotid stenosis of more than 80% was excluded from the trial. Randomization occurred in the operating room. No patient having emergent surgery or severe left ventricular dysfunction (left ventricular ejection fraction <30%) was eligible for the study. The 3 groups were nearly identical in both preoperative and operative characteristics such as sex, age, incidence of prior MI, hypertension, diabetes, pump time, and number of grafts (Table 2).

The Mathew Scale used to analyze function is an ordinate measure based on a perfect score of 100. The preoperative evaluation in each of the 3 temperature groups (cold, n = 100; tepid, n = 93; warm, n = 98) varied from 99.1 to 98.6, as close to normal as one could expect. We compared patients with their own control scores, and measured the change from preoperative to early postoperative to late follow-up. There was a significant decrease in function of 4.6% to 4.9% across all temperature groups from preoperative to immediately postoperative evaluation, with no difference noted by temperature. This initial decrease in function, in large measure, returns to normal by 1 month, but a residual depression of 1.3% to 1.8% remains, again with no distinction by temperature. This deterioration of function immediately postoperatively was found in 69% of patients, unrelated to temperature, and 48% of these patients had returned to their preoperative levels by 1 month. In all, 55% of the entire group was at or above their preoperative score at 1 month.

The 3 divisions of the neurologic evaluation—cognition, elemental skills, and disability—were examined independently and were found to individually have no correlation with the temperature of the perfusate. The neurologist determined that a stroke may have occurred in 49 of the 291 patients (17%), and a computed tomography (CT) scan was then obtained in each patient. Positive scans were found in only 13 patients (4.5%). The distribution of cerebrovascular accidents (CVAs) across temperature groups was 6 cold, 3 tepid, and 4 warm, clearly not a significant difference. Our neurologists correlated the volume of the cerebral infarct on the CT scan with the temperature of the perfusate, and there was no significant difference in the volume of infarct between temperature groups. However, it was fascinating to note that the "small" infarcts, or those less than 600 mm^3, which were the 4 lacunar, or watershed, strokes and 2 of 9 hemispheric CVAs, were not perceived as clinical abnormalities by either the surgeons, nurses, patient, or family. Thus, the perceived incidence of apparent stroke that would have been diagnosed under normal circumstances by

TABLE 2.
Clinical Data of NIH Perfusion Temperature Trial

Data	Cold	Tepid	Warm
Preoperative			
No. of patients	100	93	98
Mean age (y)	63.5 ± 0.9	62.5 ± 0.9	62.3 ± 0.9
Range of age (y)	37-75	39-75	42-75
Men (%)	7.0	78.5	80.6
Diabetes (%)	32.0	30.1	24.5
Hypertension (%)	60.0	62.4	61.2
COPD (%)	10.0	10.8	4.1
History of MI (%)	43.0	48.4	52.0
History of unstable angina (%)	62.0	62.4	62.2
Left main (%)	32.0	22.6	26.5
Operative			
No. of grafts (mean)	3.9 ± 0.1	4.0 ± 0.1	2.8 ± 0.1
Internal thoracic artery used (%)	97.0	96.8	96.0
Mean CPB time (min)	134.6 ± 4.1	139.2 ± 4.2	133.4 ± 3.8
Mean cross-clamp (min)	83.8 ± 2.8	89.2 ± 3.1	86.0 ± 3.0
Postoperative			
Perioperative mortality (%)	1.0	2.2	1.0
Peak postop weight gain (kg)	3.8 ± 1.0	3.1 ± 0.8	2.6 ± 0.3
Mean intubation time (h)	9.8 ± 0.8	8.9 ± 0.6	8.8 ± 0.6
Peak postop CK-MB level (g/L)	56.0 ± 6.7	46.4 ± 5.0	47.6 ± 4.5
Inotrope use (%)	22.0	29.0	19.4
Intra-aortic balloon pump (%)	1.0	1.1	3.1
Postoperative length of stay (d)	6.1 ± 0.4	5.3 ± 0.3	5.5 ± 0.3
Discharge within 3-5 days (%)	59.0	67.8	63.3
Range of length of stay (d)	1-21	0-21	2-20
Reoperation for bleeding (%)	0.0	1.1	4.1
Blood loss (mL)	844.3 ± 39.3	899.1 ± 44.2	961.9 ± 69.2
Patients receiving no blood products (%)	56.0	58.1	60.2
CT scan–confirmed stroke (%)	6.0	3.2	4.1
Atrial arrhythmias (%)	29.0	23.7	31.6

Abbreviations: COPD, Chronic obstructive pulmonary disease; *MI*, myocardial infarction; *CPB*, cardiopulmonary bypass; *CK-MB*, creatine kinase-MB; *CT*, computed tomography.

surgeons or nursing personnel was only 2.4% (7/291). Clearly, having a sophisticated neurologic evaluation of every patient leads to a diagnosis of more actual abnormalities than would otherwise be apparent. Not unexpectedly, increasing age was a significant ($P = .003$) predictor of worsening postoperative neurologic function, but again there was no distinction by temperature.

In this clinical trial, during warm (37°C) CPB, it was considered to be imperative for the perfusionist to maintain flow rates in excess of that which would be considered simply adequate for survival. That is to say, a bypass flow of 2.2 L/min per square meter of body surface area (BSA) might be considered by most to be appropriate.[28] We, however, established that the perfusion flow rate be maintained from 2.5 to 3.0 L/min per square meter BSA during normothermic perfusion despite increased collateral blood flow into the operative field. The maintenance of both pH and Pco_2 is considered to be a critical part of the perfusion scheme, with the pH and Pco_2 being maintained at near-normal levels by using alpha-stat blood gas management.[29]

The stabilization of systemic pressure in a nonpulsatile system is by necessity maintained with both vasodilators and vasopressors as necessary. In most circumstances, the vasodilator was simply an anesthetic gas such as isoflurane that was administered into the oxygenator at 0.5% to 2%. The vasopressor administered was usually phenylephrine (Neosynephrine).

Considerable data are now available to indicate the importance of maintaining higher systemic blood pressures for purposes of preventing hypoperfusion of vital organs, particularly the brain.[30] In the presence of CPB, cerebral perfusion distal to any atherosclerotic lesion is pressure dependent. The risk of central nervous system (CNS) injury can be directly reflective of the adequacy of mean systemic blood pressure for preventing CNS dysfunction. Basically, our group therefore maintained the patient's mean blood pressure during CPB at the level of the patient's mean blood pressure when he is resting normally. This would mean that a hypertensive patient with a mean blood pressure in the range of 90 to 100 mm Hg would be maintained at a comparable mean blood pressure level during bypass. Hypertensive patients who normally have mean blood pressures above 100 mm Hg are at increased risk of postoperative cerebral dysfunction and are clearly more likely to have a lacunar or watershed infarct.

Only in recent years have surgeons begun to use perfusion temperatures that are considered to be "warm." Most commonly, perfusion had been performed at temperatures less than 30°C. Although hypothermia is clearly one of the most effective measures to protect the brain when it is likely to become ischemic, there is the downside to hypothermia, namely the necessity for rewarming.

There can be no debate about the adverse consequences of cerebral hyperthermia.[31] Hyperthermia to 39°C increases cerebral ischemia, leading to infarction in the potentially ischemic brain.[7] Because the rewarming process during CPB is an integral part of hypothermic perfusion, raising cerebral temperature may potentiate ischemia and even lead to infarction.[7] In fact, with rewarming, the cerebral metabolic demand may exceed brain oxygen delivery, resulting in the clinical finding of increased extraction and jugular venous desaturation.[8] For a period of several hours after rewarming, there may be a cerebral demand for increased oxygen and glucose extraction because the CBF may not increase sufficiently to meet the increased demand.[32] This suggests a vulnerable period for cerebral ischemia during and after rewarming when increased CBF could be the limiting factor in preventing ischemic infarction. Newman et al[33] have documented how increasing the rapidity of rewarming is associated with cognitive dysfunction in the elderly.

An additional feature of CNS metabolic function related to temperature concerns glutamate, a major excitatory neurotransmitter and a potent neurotoxin.[34] The extracellular concentration of glutamate is tightly regulated under normal conditions by the reuptake of released glutamate. There is an excitotoxic theory of ischemic neuronal injury which proposes that ischemia leads to the increased release and impaired uptake of glutamate. The elevation in extracellular glutamate leads to activation of N-methyl-D-aspartate (NMDA) and amino-3 hydroxy-5-methyl-4-isoxazolepropionate (AMPA) receptors, an influx of Ca^{2+} into the cell, and a cascade of events leading to cell death.[35] Even mild hypothermia of 33°C reduces the increase in extracellular glutamate occurring during ischemia.[36] This is an additional factor in support of tepid rather than normothermic perfusion.

Neurologic dysfunction after bypass is believed to result from 4 possible etiologies: (1) macroembolization of particulate matter, gas, atheromata, or thrombus; (2) microembolization of gas, fat, or plastic particles, and microaggregates of platelets, cells, and fibrin; (3) inadequate cerebral capillary perfusion from the influence of CPB (eg, sludging of blood); and (4) inadequate cerebral perfusion as a result of reduced flow, reduced perfusion pressure, or both.[37,38]

Cerebral embolization can be readily documented with noninvasive Doppler ultrasound used during CPB.[38] In fact, most emboli have been shown to occur on initiation of CPB, manipulation of the ascending aorta, and when the heart resumes ejecting at the completion of CPB.[39] Numerous studies document that the neuropsychological disturbance frequently occurring in patients post-

CPB is a consequence of diffuse cerebral embolization.[39,40] Watershed or lacunar infarcts may be suggestive of global cerebral hypoperfusion, but even in these conditions cerebral embolization cannot be ruled out.[41] Hypothermia is beneficial in a setting of transient ischemia, such as may occur with regional hypoperfusion in the presence of cerebral vascular disease. However, most intraoperative strokes are probably caused by cerebral embolization that produces permanent, not transient ischemia.[42,43] There can be no reason to expect hypothermia to be totally protective in this setting.[42] However, because the use of mild hypothermia during CPB (even a 3°C to 4°C decrease in temperature) confers significant protection in the setting of transient ischemia, it is reasonable to expect a tepid perfusion temperature to decrease the severity of neurologic dysfunction even in the setting of a permanent, limited focal deficit.[43] This is the main argument for allowing the perfusion temperature to drift during CPB, allowing the temperature to reach 32°C to 34°C before warming gradually.

INFLAMMATORY RESPONSE TO CPB

CPB by definition involves extracorporeal circulation and the resultant activation of inflammatory mediators and blood elements. These inflammatory compounds induce endothelial injury that is often cell mediated and can lead to myocardial and respiratory dysfunction. Although myocardial reperfusion injury may be one manifestation of this response, such injury has been classically attributed to calcium homeostasis at the cellular level. The exposure of blood to the artificial surfaces inherent in extracorporeal circulation induces an acute inflammatory response that is well known to surgeons.[44] This inflammatory response may be associated with morbidity and, in fact, can often result in organ dysfunction. The inflammatory mediators activated by extracorporeal circulation include complement, neutrophils, mononuclear cells, and platelets, all of which can lead to cytokine release.[45-47] The activation of neutrophils is associated with CPB, leading to their adhesion to endothelial cells, followed by transendothelial migration and the release of neutrophil-derived cytotoxic products, in particular oxygen-free radicals and proteolytic enzymes (Figs 1-3).[48,49]

We feel certain that neutrophils are a primary factor in the inflammatory response elicited by extracorporeal circulation and may be responsible for the development of postoperative organ dysfunction.[50,51] The issue to be addressed concerns whether this

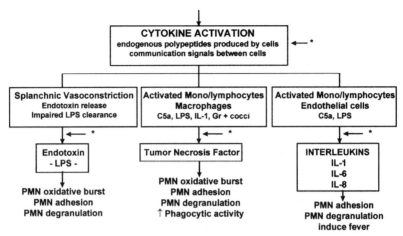

FIGURE 1.
Cardiopulmonary bypass induces an inflammatory state manifested by cytokine generation and activation of blood cells, which incite a noxious response. *Abbreviations: LPS,* Lipopolysaccharide; *IL,* interleukin; *Gr +,* gram-positive; *PMN,* polymorphonuclear neutrophil.

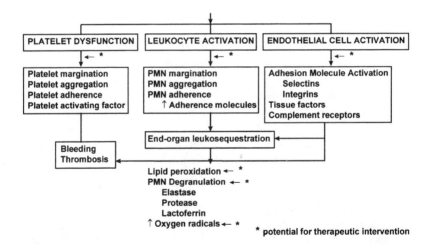

FIGURE 2.
The inflammatory state involves a cellular cascade, predominately manifesting endothelial and leukocyte activation and platelet dysfunction. These changes result in generation of adherence molecules and tissue factors, with extravasation of leukocytes into the extravascular tissue. In addition, platelet activation leads to margination and adherence of the platelets to the endothelium. Potential sites of therapeutic intervention are indicated by an *asterisk. Abbreviation: PMN,* Polymorphonuclear neutrophil.

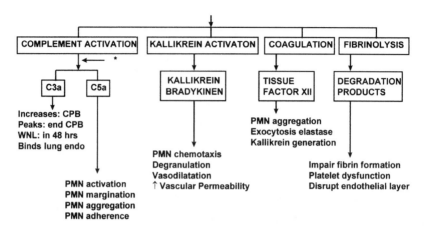

* potential for therapeutic intervention

FIGURE 3.

The inflammatory state includes a humoral cascade with products generated within the bloodstream. These include complement, kallikreins, and both coagulation and fibrinolytic factors. These factors cause systemic reactions that can be noxious. *Abbreviations: CPB,* Cardiopulmonary bypass; *WNL,* within normal limits; *endo,* endothelium; *PMN,* polymorphonuclear neutrophil.

inflammatory response can be influenced by intraoperative CPB perfusion temperature.

The schemata for generation of inflammatory elements are illustrated in Figures 1 to 3. There is the overall effect of bypass on inducing cytokine activation, which, although reduced at hypothermia, is clearly increased after rewarming (Fig 1).[52,53] Figures 2 and 3 document the cellular and humoral cascades that function through unique pathways, yet remarkably yield the same end result—polymorphonuclear degranulation with release of protease, elastase, and oxygen-free radicals. These toxic products lead to membrane and endothelial degradation with increased vascular permeability and end-organ leukosequestration. Ultimately, respiratory organ dysfunction becomes a factor in patient recovery, and it is appropriate to consider whether perfusion temperature is also a factor. The data as presented to date suggest that temperature is not a major determinant in the development of the inflammatory condition seen after CPB.[52,53] Although the release of inflammatory mediators is reduced while hypothermic, the reversal of perfusion requires a rewarming process that leads ultimately to the same inflammatory condition present after warm CPB.

FIBRINOLYIC ACTIVITY AFTER CPB

The schematic for the activation and inhibition of fibrinolysis during CPB is illustrated in Figure 4. The contact of blood with artificial surfaces leads to the activation of Hageman factor (factor XII) and the conversion of prekallikrein to kallikrein.[54] Both actions serve to degrade plasminogen to plasmin. Additionally, activated factor XII initiates the clotting cascade by promoting the formation of thrombin from prothrombin. During CPB, the endothelial cell is

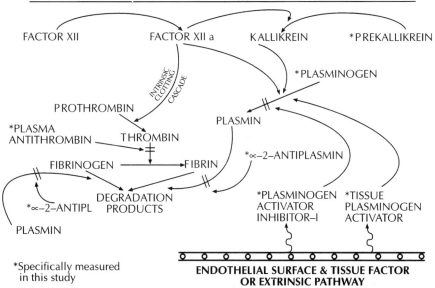

ARTIFICIAL SURFACE & CPB CONTACT ACTIVATION OR INTRINSIC PATHWAY

*Specifically measured in this study

ENDOTHELIAL SURFACE & TISSUE FACTOR OR EXTRINSIC PATHWAY

FIGURE 4.

A schematic for fibrinolytic potential occurring during cardiopulmonary bypass *(CPB)*. Blood and artificial surface contact lead to activation of Hageman factor (factor XII) and conversion of prekallikrein to kallikrein. Both serve to degrade plasminogen into plasmin. Plasmin actively degrades fibrin, producing fibrinolysis. Activated factor XII, also through its initiation of the clotting cascade, promotes formation of thrombin from prothrombin. Disturbances during CPB may affect the endothelial cell and thereby promote formation of tissue plasminogen activator (t-PA), which functions to support the degradation of plasminogen to plasmin and an antifibrinolytic, plasminogen activator inhibitor-1 (PAI-1). The latter functions to interrupt the degradation of plasminogen to plasmin. Specifically measured and reported in the text are those products marked with an *asterisk*, t-PA antigen, PAI-1, plasma antithrombin, plasminogen, prekallikrein, and α-2-antiplasmin. (Courtesy of Engelman RM, Pleet AB, Rousou JA, et al: The influence of cardiopulmonary bypass (CPB) perfusion temperature on neurologic and hematologic function after coronary artery bypass grafting (CABG). *Ann Thorac Surg* 67:1547-1556, 1999. Reprinted with permission from the Society of Thoracic Surgeons.)

affected by both myocardial ischemia and cardioplegia, contributing to the generation of the fibrinolytic, tissue plasminogen activator (t-PA) antigen, and the antifibrinolytic or prothrombotic, plasminogen activator inhibitor-1 (PAI-1).[55-57] While t-PA functions to support the degradation of plasminogen to plasmin, PAI-1 functions to interrupt this degradation. When both t-PA and PAI-1 are generated, the former is more physiologically dominant, meaning the potential for fibrinolytic activity is greater.[58]

We performed, as part of this NIH-funded trial, a randomized prospective hematologic study in 53 patients undergoing coronary revascularization at either normothermic (37°C), tepid (32°C), or hypothermic (20°C) perfusion. In this study, 6 different hematologic parameters were measured before bypass, immediately after completion of CPB, and intermittently for the first 24 hours of recovery. The measured parameters (illustrated with an asterisk in Fig 4) were t-PA, PAI-1, and plasma antithrombin, plasminogen, prekallikrein, and α_2-antiplasmin. As can be seen in Figure 4, the role of each of these hematologic factors in the fibrinolytic system is clearly defined. The actual results, corrected for hemodilution and expressed as a percent of the preoperative determination, are described in Table 3, comparing the immediate postoperative study with the preoperative evaluation. The analyses document that plasminogen and prekallikrein levels decrease as a percent of the preoperative controls only in the tepid and warm patients. There was a trend to a decreasing plasminogen and prekallikrein level with increasing temperature. This decrease is consistent with the degradation of plasminogen to plasmin and prekallikrein to kallikrein (Fig 4).

The presence of a temperature-dependent effect on plasminogen and prekallikrein supports the conclusion that artificial surface–induced fibrinolysis is temperature dependent, and that normothermic perfusion leads to increased fibrinolytic potential. On the other hand, the absence of a correlation with temperature regarding the endothelial-generated factors of t-PA and PAI-1 implies that there is no increased endothelial stimulation at normothermia compared with hypothermia.

The postoperative clinical data of the 291 patients divided into the 3 groups is illustrated in Table 2. The effects of warm perfusion were associated with the highest blood loss, but the difference was not statistically significant. The cold group had no reoperations for bleeding, whereas the warm group had a 4.1% reoperative rate ($0.1 > P > .05$). Patients in the tepid group had only a 1.1% incidence of reoperation. This study has shown that normothermic perfusion leads to increased fibrinolysis. Tepid perfusion clearly is

TABLE 3.

Summary Data for Hematologic Studies: Percent Change From
Preoperative Levels

Test	Temp	Mean	SE	Trend
PAT	Cold	1.2	4.4	$P = .14$
	Tepid	6.3	6.2	
	Warm	−4.4	8.3	
	All	0.8	4.0	
A2	Cold	8.5	5.0	$P = .24$
	Tepid	7.8	7.2	
	Warm	1.2	9.4	
	All	5.5	4.5	
PLS	Cold	6.5	6.4	$P = .06$
	Tepid	−4.4	7.0	
	Warm	−5.3	9.6	
	All	−1.8	4.7	
t-PA	Cold	162.2	26.5	$P = .96$
	Tepid	155.5	34.4	
	Warm	203.2	49.5	
	All	175.8	23.3	
PK	Cold	4.0	6.7	$P = .02$
	Tepid	−3.2	6.6	
	Warm	−13.7	9.0	
	All	−5.3	4.6	
PAI-1	Cold	3855	334	$P = .981$
	Tepid	4373	408	
	Warm	402	133	
	All	2670	1519	

Abbreviations: Temp, Temperature; *PAT,* plasma antithrombin III; *A2,* α-2-antiplasmin; *PLS,* plasminogen; *t-PA,* tissue plasminogen activator; *PK,* prekallikrein; *PAI-1,* plasminogen activator inhibitor-1.

an improvement in terms of fibrinolytic potential and is therefore the recommended temperature rather than normothermic perfusion.

INFLUENCE OF TEMPERATURE ON PULMONARY AND SYSTEMIC EFFECTS OF CPB

The influence of perfusion temperature on postoperative pulmonary function is clearly dependent on the presence or absence of hypothermia in the postoperative patient. Rewarming frequently causes an afterdrop in the early recovery phase, which simply means the body temperature has not equilibrated and the core temperature may be 32°C to 34°C. This makes extubation difficult and may impair pulmonary gas exchange. Two studies were recently conducted in hypothermic and normothermic patients with[59] and without[60] compromised pulmonary function. In the study conducted in patients with preoperative abnormal lung function,[59] the alveolar-arterial oxygen levels showed a lower gradient, or better function, in the normothermic group immediately postoperatively that equalized at 3 hours. The incidence of postextubation pulmonary dysfunction was lower in the normothermic group (12% vs 44%). In the study conducted in patients with uncompromised lung function, the alveolar-arterial gradients were identical in the hypothermic and normothermic patients.

Perfusion temperature has been studied in its relationship to renal function.[61] In a prospective randomized trial of hypothermic, tepid, and warm perfusion, glomerular and tubular renal function were assessed. No difference was apparent between the 3 temperature groups, and the authors concluded that perfusion temperature has no influence on renal function in patients having coronary bypass grafting.

Two studies[62,63] have investigated the effect of temperature on gastric and intestinal mucosal perfusion during and after CPB. Both studies[62,63] were randomized trials that used hypothermic (28°C to 30°C) or tepid/normothermic (35°C to 37°C) perfusion. Both used tonometry measurements for determining gastric pH, and one study[63] measured gastric wall blood flow with a laser Doppler device. In both studies, the influence of CPB temperature was of little import on mucosal perfusion, with other overriding factors contributing to any mucosal hypoxia. There is a significant reduction in pH after CPB, indicating possible hypoxia regardless of perfusion temperature, and no difference was noted between hypothermic and normothermic patients.[62,63]

PARAMETERS OF ADEQUATE PERFUSION

It is our impression that perfusion temperature is best maintained at a tepid level of 32°C to 34°C. This level provides an adequate temperature for cerebral protection while permitting effective and rapid rewarming without inciting hyperthermia. In fact, the best approach is to allow the perfusion temperature to drift down, which it will do in our cool operating suites. Warming is initiated when the core temperature reaches 32°C to 34°C, and rewarming is gradually accomplished, as the cessation of bypass is contemplated, in 15 to 30 minutes. Hyperthermia is avoided.

The flow rate is maintained near 2.5 L/min per square meter BSA, and perfusion pressure is maintained near the patient's normal preoperative mean blood pressure. Hypotension is avoided, and both the initiation and the discontinuation of CPB are performed gradually. Maintaining an adequate perfusion pressure is essential in the nonpulsatile hemodiluted environment of CPB. Given these parameters, a safe pump run is achieved within the time frame necessary to perform even the most complex operations.

The acid-base management during CPB is best conducted via alpha-stat regulation.[29] Often we have found that our tepid/normothermic patients who are normothermic after bypass have a metabolic acidosis, which has not been a concern. This responds to sodium bicarbonate administration and does not delay extubation. The explanation for even a transient metabolic acidosis must rest with inadequacies of nonpulsatile perfusion. Because this acidosis is uniformly benign and easily corrected, we have not studied its pathogenesis or attempted to alter our perfusion techniques. Previously, when patients were hypothermic postbypass, not only was acidosis a problem, but also peripheral vasoconstriction was evident secondary to a decreased core temperature. Now vasodilatation is most common with high cardiac outputs.

In summary, we recommend:

1. Tepid perfusion allowing temperature to drift to 32°C to 34°C
2. Flow rates of 2.2 to 2.5 L/min per square meter BSA with a perfusion pressure adjusted to the patient's normal mean pressure
3. Alpha-stat pH management
4. Avoidance of hyperthermia
5. Gradual changes in perfusion flows and pressures rather than abrupt alterations.

REFERENCES

1. Lichtenstein SV, El Dalati H, Panos A, et al: Long cross-clamp times with warm heart surgery. *Lancet* 1:1443-1444, 1989.
2. O'Dwyer C, Prough DS, Johnston WE: Determinants of cerebral perfusion during cardiopulmonary bypass. *J Cardiothorac Vasc Anesth* 10:54-65, 1996.
3. Bigelow WG, Kindsay WK, Greenwood WF: Hypothermia: Its possible role in cardiac surgery in an investigation of factors governing survival in dogs at low body temperatures. *Ann Surg* 132:849-866, 1950.
4. Ginsberg MD, Stemau LL, Globus MY, et al: Therapeutic modulation of brain temperature: Relevance to ischemic brain injury. *Cerebrovasc Brain Metab Rev* 4:189-225, 1992.

5. Croughwell N, Smith LR, Quill T, et al: The effect of temperature on cerebral metabolism and blood flow in adults during cardiopulmonary bypass. *J Thorac Cardiovasc Surg* 103:549-554, 1992.

6. Taylor RH, Burrow FA, Bissonnette B: Cerebral pressure-flow velocity relationship during hypothermic cardiopulmonary bypass in neonates and infants. *Anesth Analg* 74:636-642, 1992.

7. Ginsberg MD, Globus MY, Dietrich WD, et al: Temperature modulation of ischemic brain injury: A synthesis of recent advances. *Prog Brain Res* 96:13-22, 1993.

8. Cook DJ, Oliver WC Jr, Orzulak TA, et al: A prospective randomized comparison of cerebral venous oxygen saturation during normothermic and hypothermic cardiopulmonary bypass. *J Thorac Cardiovasc Surg* 107:1020-1029, 1994.

9. McLean J: The thromboplastic action of cephalin. *Am J Physiol* 41:250-257, 1916.

10. Chargaff E, Olson K: Studies on the chemistry of blood coagulation: V1. Studies on the action of heparin and other anticoagulations: The influence of protamine on the anticoagulant effect in vivo. *J Biol Chem* 122:153-167, 1937.

11. Dale HH, Schuster EHJ: A double perfusion pump. *J Physiol* 64:356-364, 1928.

12. Debakey ME: Simple continuous-flow blood transfusion instrument. *New Orleans Med Soc* 87:386-389, 1934.

13. Dennis C, Spreng DS, Nelson GE, et al: Development of a pump-oxygenator to replace the heart and lungs: An apparatus applicable to human patients and an application to one case. *Ann Surg* 134:709-721, 1951.

14. DeWall RA: A simple expandable artificial oxygenator for open heart surgery. *Surg Clin North Am* 36:1025-1034, 1956.

15. Drinker PA, Bartlett RH, Mialer AM, et al: Augmentation of membrane gas transfer by induced secondary flows. *Surgery* 66:775-781, 1969.

16. Bodell BR, Head JM, Head LR: A capillary membrane oxygenator. *J Thorac Cardiovasc Surg* 46:639-650, 1963.

17. Rafferty EH, Kletschka HD, Olsen DA: A nonpulsatile artificial heart. *J Extracorp Tech* 5:6-11, 1973.

18. Dennis C: Perspective in review: One groups struggle with development of a pump-oxygenator. *Trans Am Soc Artif Intern Organs* 31:1-11, 1985.

19. Lillehei CS: Historical development of cardiopulmonary bypass, in Gravlee GP, David RF, Utley JR (eds): *Cardiopulmonary Bypass: Principles and Practice.* Baltimore, Md, Williams & Wilkins, 1993, pp 1-26.

20. Zuhdi N, McCollough B, Carey J, et al: Hypothermic perfusion for open heart surgical procedures. *J Int Coll Surg* 35:319-325, 1961.

21. Shumway NE, Lower RR, Stofer RC: Selective hypothermia of the heart in anoxic cardiac arrest. *Surg Gynecol Obstet* 109:750-754, 1959.

22. Buckberg GD, Brazier J, Nelson RL: Studies of the effects of hypothermia on regional myocardial blood flow and metabolism during cardiopulmonary bypass: I. The adequately perfused, beating, fibrillating, and arrested heart. *J Thorac Cardiovasc Surg* 78:87-94, 1977.
23. Lichtenstein SV, Ashe KA, Dalati HE: Warm heart surgery. *J Thorac Cardiovasc Surg* 101:269-274, 1991.
24. Hearse DJ, Stewart DA, Braimbridge MV: The additive protective effects of hypothermia and chemical cardioplegia during ischemic cardiac arrest in the dog. *J Thorac Cardiovasc Surg* 79:29-38, 1980.
25. Kirklin JW, Barratt-Boyes BG: *Cardiac Surgery*, ed 2. New York, Churchill Livingstone, 1992, pp 61-91.
26. Cook DJ, Oliver WC Jr, Orzulak TA, et al: Cardiopulmonary bypass temperature, hematocrit, and cerebral oxygen delivery in humans. *Ann Thorac Surg* 60:1671-1677, 1995.
27. Engelman RM, Pleet AB, Rousou JA, et al: The influence of cardiopulmonary bypass (CPB) perfusion temperature on neurologic and hematologic function after coronary artery bypass grafting (CABG). *Ann Thorac Surg* 67:1547-1556, 1999.
28. Robiscek F, Masters GN, Niesluchowski W, et al: Vasomotor activity during cardiopulmonary bypass, in Utley JR (ed): *Pathophysiology and Techniques of Cardiopulmonary Bypass*, vol 2. Baltimore, Md, Williams & Wilkins, 1983.
29. Tallman RD: Acid-base regulation, alpha-state, and the emperor's new clothes. *J Cardiothorac Vasc Anesth* 11:282-288, 1997.
30. Gold J, Krieger KB, Isom OW: Improvement of outcomes after coronary artery bypass. *J Thorac Cardiovasc Surg* 110:1304-1314, 1995.
31. Miyazawa T, Bonnekoh P, Widmann R: Heating of the brain to maintain normothermia during ischemia aggravates brain injury in the rat. *Acta Neuropathol* 85:488-494, 1993.
32. Mezrow CK, Sadeghi AM, Gandsas A: Cerebral blood flow and metabolism in hypothermic circulatory arrest. *Ann Thorac Surg* 54:609-616, 1992.
33. Newman MF, Kramer D, Croughwell ND, et al: Differential age effects of mean artificial pressure and rewarming on cognitive dysfunction after cardiac surgery. *Anesth Analg* 81:236-242, 1995.
34. Nakashima T, Todd MM: The effect of hypothermia on the rate of excitatory amino acids release after cerebral ischemia. *Anesthesiology* 81:815A, 1994.
35. Foster AC, Gill R, Iversen LL: Therapeutic potential of NMDA receptor antagonists as neuroprotective agents. *Prog Clin Biol Res* 361:301-329, 1990.
36. Ginsberg MD, Stemau LL, Globus MY-T: Therapeutic modulation of brain temperature: Relevance to ischemic brain injury. *Cerebrovasc Brain Metab Rev* 4:189-225, 1992.
37. Mills SA, Prough DS: Neuropsychiatric complications following cardiac surgery. *Semin Thorac Cardiovasc Surg* 3:39-46, 1991.

38. Hindman BJ: Neurologic complications of cardiac anesthesia and surgery. *Curr Opin Anaesth* 6:93-97, 1993.

39. Mills SA: Cerebral injury and cardiac operations. *Ann Thorac Surg* 46:86S-91S, 1993.

40. Pugsley W, Klinger L, Paschalis C, et al: Microemboli and cerebral impairment during cardiac surgery. *Vasc Surg* 24:34-43, 1990.

41. Torvik A: The pathogenesis of watershed infarcts in the brain. *Stroke* 15:221-223, 1984.

42. Ridenour TR, Warner DS, Todd MM: Mild hypothermia reduces infarct size resulting from temporary but not permanent focal ischemia in rats. *Stroke* 23:733-738, 1992.

43. McLean RF, Wong BI: Normothermic versus hypothermic cardiopulmonary bypass: Central nervous system outcomes. *J Cardiothorac Vasc Anesth* 10:45-53, 1996.

44. Westaby S: Organ dysfunction after cardiopulmonary bypass: A systemic inflammatory reaction initiated by the extracorporeal circuit. *Intensive Care Med* 13:89-95, 1987.

45. Kirklin IK, Westaby S, Blackstone EH, et al: Complements and the damaging effects of cardiopulmonary bypass. *J Thorac Cardiovasc Surg* 86:845-857, 1983.

46. Butler J, Rocker GM, Westaby S: Inflammatory response to cardiopulmonary bypass. *Ann Thorac Surg* 55:552-559, 1993.

47. Butler J, Chong GL, Baigrie RJ, et al: Cytokine responses to cardiopulmonary bypass with membrane and bubble oxygenation. *Ann Thorac Surg* 53:833-838, 1992.

48. Elliott MJ, Finn AHR: Interaction between neutrophils and endothelium. *Ann Thorac Surg* 56:1503-1508, 1993.

49. Shappell SB, Toman C, Anderson DC, et al: Mac-1 (CDllb/CD18) mediates adherence-dependent hydrogen peroxide production by human and canine neutrophils. *J Immunol* 44:2702-2711, 1990.

50. Taggart DP, E1-Fiky M, Carater R, et al: Respiratory dysfunction after uncomplicated cardiopulmonary bypass. *Ann Thorac Surg* 56:1123-1128, 1993.

51. Seghaye MC, Duchateau J, Grabitz RG, et al: Complement activation during cardiopulmonary bypass in infants and children: Relation to postoperative multisystem organ failure. *J Thorac Cardiovasc Surg* 106:978-987, 1993.

52. Finn A, Naik S, Klein N, et al: Interleukin-8 release and neutrophil degranulation after pediatric cardiopulmonary bypass. *J Thorac Cardiovasc Surg* 105:2324-2341, 1993.

53. Jansen NJ, van Oeveren W, Gu YJ, et al: Endotoxin release and tumor necrosis factor formation during cardiopulmonary bypass. *Ann Thorac Surg* 54:744-748, 1992.

54. Holloway DS, Summaria L, Sandesara J, et al: Decreased platelet number and function and increased fibrinolysis contribute to postoperative bleeding in cardiopulmonary bypass patients. *Thromb Haemost* 59:62-67, 1988.

55. Tanaka K, Takao M, Yada I, et al: Alteration in coagulation and fibrinolysis associated with cardiopulmonary bypass during open heart surgery. *J Cardiothorac Anesth* 3:181-188, 1989.
56. Gram S, Janetzko T, Jespersen J, et al: Enhanced effective fibrinolysis following the neutralization of heparin in open heart surgery increases the risk of post-surgical bleeding. *Thromb Haemost* 63:241-245, 1990.
57. Valen G, Eriksson E, Risberg B, et al: Fibrinolysis during cardiac surgery. *Eur J Cardiothorac Surg* 8:324-330, 1994.
58. Zilla P, yon Oppell U, Deutsch M: The endothelium: A key to the future. *J Card Surg* 8:32-60, 1993.
59. Ranucci M, Soro G, Frigiola A, et al: Normothermic perfusion and lung function after cardiopulmonary bypass: Effects in pulmonary risk patients. *Perfusion* 12:309-315, 1997.
60. Birdi I, Regragui IA, Izzat MB, et al: Effects of cardiopulmonary bypass temperature on pulmonary gas exchange after coronary artery operations. *Ann Thorac Surg* 61:118-123, 1996.
61. Regragui IA, Izzat MB, Birdi I, et al: Cardiopulmonary bypass perfusion temperature does not influence perioperative renal function. *Ann Thorac Surg* 60:160-164, 1995.
62. Croughwell ND, Newman MF, Lowry RD, et al: Effect of temperature during cardiopulmonary bypass on gastric mucosal perfusion. *Br J Anaesth* 78:34-38, 1997.
63. Ohri SK, Bowles CW, Mathie RT, et al: Effect of cardiopulmonary bypass perfusion protocols on gut tissue oxygenation and blood flow. *Ann Thorac Surg* 64:163-170, 1997.

CHAPTER 8

Pediatric Interventional Cardiology: The Cardiologist's Role and Relationship With Pediatric Cardiothoracic Surgery

David J. Waight, MD
Assistant Professor of Clinical Pediatrics, Section of Pediatric
Cardiology, Pritzker School of Medicine, University of Chicago
Children's Hospital

Ziyad M. Hijazi, MD, MPH
Professor of Pediatrics and Medicine, Section of Pediatric Cardiology,
Pritzker School of Medicine; Chief, Section of Pediatric Cardiology,
University of Chicago Children's Hospital

Pediatric cardiologists and congenital heart surgeons have worked together from the inception of pediatric cardiac surgery to optimize the preoperative management and plan the operative procedures required for patients with congenital heart disease (CHD). Pediatric cardiologists have been using cardiac catheterization and angiography for more than 4 decades. For much of that time, the anatomical and hemodynamic information obtained during cardiac catheterization had been the gold standard for the diagnosis of CHD. In the 21st century, the advanced imaging and physiologic data obtainable with echocardiography and magnetic resonance imaging have largely replaced cardiac catheterization for diagnostic and surgical planning indications. The pediatric catheterization laboratories have become increasingly used for interventional treatment of CHD.

The relationship between pediatric cardiology and cardiothoracic surgery has evolved as advancements in the surgical management of complex CHD have resulted in the survival of most patients. These patients often require staging of their repairs, resulting in surgical difficulties because of multiple operations. Rapid development of successful interventional procedures in the 1980s and 1990s has led to interventional procedures becoming the primary treatment of many forms of heart disease. Interventional procedures have also become essential in the optimal staging of the surgical management of patients with complex anatomy. The interventional cardiologist and the congenital heart surgeon must both understand the other's capabilities to offer the optimal treatment of common problems and the appropriate single therapy or staged repair of complex disorders.

In this chapter, currently available pediatric interventional catheterization procedures and their relation to cardiothoracic surgery are discussed. Investigational procedures are also discussed, and expected future developments are introduced. The goal of this chapter is to provide the congenital heart surgeon with a reference for the available alternatives to surgical repair of CHD and to discuss how interventional procedures can be incorporated into the surgical management of complex CHD.

ATRIAL SEPTOSTOMY
BALLOON ATRIOSEPTOSTOMY

The management of patients that require intra-atrial mixing of fully oxygenated and venous blood has improved since the introduction of balloon atrioseptostomy in 1966. This was the first interventional procedure in pediatric cardiology and also the first coordinated staged repair, with interventional cardiology providing a temporizing procedure until a definitive cardiothoracic surgical repair could be performed.[1] Balloon atrioseptostomy can be indicated in the management of patients with transposition of the great arteries, tricuspid atresia, pulmonary atresia, mitral atresia, and total anomalous pulmonary venous return. The transcatheter atrioseptostomy procedure has changed little since its inception. The enlarged atrial septal defect (ASD) allows improved mixing and an improved cardiac output or systemic oxygenation. Many institutions perform atrioseptostomies at the bedside in the neonatal nursery under echocardiographic guidance.[2] The reported mortality is 0.7% and the success rate is 99%.[3] In general, balloon atrioseptostomy is limited to the first month of life because the intra-atrial septum becomes thickened and the balloon fails to tear the septum.

BLADE ATRIOSEPTOSTOMY

Older patients can be effectively palliated with blade atrial septostomy as described by Park et al[4,5] in 1975. This procedure entails passing a retractable cutting blade across the atrial septum through a patent foramen ovale or through a transseptal puncture site, opening the blade, and pulling the blade across the septum. Patients at any age are candidates for this procedure. In addition to the above indications, blade septostomy can be useful in the management of patients with severe pulmonary hypertension. By creating an ASD, the patients have improved cardiac output, but do become slightly cyanotic because of the right-to-left shunting. The improved cardiac output may relieve or improve the patient's symptoms and may be used as a bridge to lung transplantation.[6]

STATIC BALLOON DILATION

Newborns with hypoplastic left heart syndrome or other complex cyanotic heart disease who are awaiting heart transplant may eventually develop a severely restrictive ASD. They develop pulmonary venous hypertension and pulmonary edema, and become progressively cyanotic. Standard balloon atrioseptostomy can be effective, but creates an unrestricted ASD that can lead to high oxygen saturations and a low systemic cardiac output state in patients with hypoplastic left heart syndrome. These patients can be effectively palliated with static balloon dilation of their ASD. This palliative procedure can be repeated until a suitable organ becomes available for transplantation.

These techniques for ASD creation can also be applied to patients who may benefit from an intra-atrial shunt, such as those with right or left ventricular dysfunction. The ASD then allows decompression of the high-pressure atrial chamber. Patients receiving extracorporeal membrane oxygenation because of left ventricular dysfunction have been shown to benefit from ASD creation, with possible return of normal left ventricular function or as a bridge to heart transplantation.[7]

BALLOON VALVULOPLASTY
PULMONARY VALVULOPLASTY

Kan et al[8] reported the first transcatheter balloon valvuloplasty in 1982. The technique involves passing a balloon dilation catheter antegrade over a wire across the pulmonary valve. The balloon is then inflated to its maximum size, which is selected as 100% to 120% of the size of the pulmonary valve annulus. The procedure is repeated 2 to 4 times for less than 10 to 15 seconds per inflation. Balloon pulmonary valvuloplasty has uniformly excellent results in infants, children, and adults. It has a low recurrence risk and can be easily repeated if necessary. This has become the procedure of choice for the treatment of isolated pulmonary valve stenosis in any institution with the proper facilities.[9-11] The same techniques have been applied to infants with critical pulmonary stenosis who require emergent intervention or a prostaglandin infusion to maintain ductal patency. The success rate is less in this patient group, with 6% to 23% of procedures unsuccessful.[12-14] These patients then require a surgical valvotomy. A comparison of surgical and transcatheter approaches demonstrated that the transcatheter treatment group had a lower mortality than did the surgical valvotomy group. This has led many to use transcatheter balloon valvuloplasty as the first-line therapy for critical pulmonary stenosis.

PULMONARY ATRESIA AND INTACT VENTRICULAR SEPTUM

Patients with pulmonary atresia and an intact ventricular septum have commonly required a staged procedure with initial palliation with a modified Blalock-Taussig shunt (BTS) and right ventricular outflow tract patch. Many of these patients are now initially palliated in the interventional cardiac catheterization laboratory. Several techniques for perforating the atretic pulmonary valve have been used successfully to allow balloon pulmonary valvotomy. The stiff end of a guidewire may be used to create a small hole in the valve plate, which is then crossed with the floppy end of the wire.[15] Radiofrequency ablation catheters or laser perforation have also been used to perforate the pulmonary valve plate. This is done as a retrograde or antegrade technique, which then allows passage of a guidewire and then a balloon catheter for balloon valvuloplasty.[16-20] The early worldwide results with these techniques demonstrate a combined success rate of 79.7% and a mortality of 4.3%.[21] A number of these patients may require prolonged prostaglandin infusions to maintain ductal patency and provide a second source of pulmonary blood flow. Some patients will still require a BTS because of continued severe cyanosis.

Transcatheter palliation in patients with pulmonary atresia and an intact ventricular septum has also been performed with stent placement in the patent ductus arteriosus (PDA).[21] This provides a stable source of pulmonary arterial blood flow until further surgical intervention is performed.

There is an incidence of recurrent narrowing of the right ventricular outflow tract in both balloon valvuloplasty and surgical valvuloplasty, despite improvement in the right ventricular size. Transcatheter balloon valvuloplasty is then the indicated procedure and has demonstrated good results.[22,23] When the right ventricular output becomes adequate, a BTS becomes unnecessary and can be closed in the catheterization laboratory (see Occlusion Devices section).

AORTIC VALVULOPLASTY

Aortic balloon valvuloplasty was initially reported in 1984, and because of its safety and efficacy, this transcatheter technique has become the primary intervention in most centers.[24,25] Balloon aortic valvotomy is limited to patients with mild or absent aortic insufficiency and has had poor results in patients with unicommissural valves. The recent use of a carotid artery cutdown to create a direct course to the aortic valve has demonstrated improved success rates and allowed shorter procedure times in neonates with critical aortic stenosis.[26,27] This cutdown procedure reflects coordination between interventionalist and surgeon that is frequently continued in patients with aortic valve stenosis who may need further intervention. A more coordinated cooperation has been described with transventricular balloon dilation of critical aortic stenosis. This procedure allows balloon dilation of the stenotic valve in the operating room without requiring cardiopulmonary bypass, but can be converted to an open aortic valvuloplasty if necessary.[28,29]

Balloon aortic valvuloplasty may be repeated in approximately 30% of patients who have restenosis, as long as the aortic insufficiency is no worse than mild. A smaller percentage of patients (17%-27%) eventually require surgical valvotomy, valve replacement, or a Ross procedure.[30,31]

MITRAL AND TRICUSPID VALVULOPLASTY

The incidence of congenital mitral or tricuspid valve stenosis is very low, and these malformations are frequently associated with other CHD. Rheumatic disease leading to stenosis of the atrioventricular valves has occasionally been observed in children. There has been a large experience with balloon dilation of the mitral valve in adults with rheumatic heart disease, with less experience in children.

ANGIOPLASTY AND STENTS
PULMONARY ARTERY STENOSIS

Branch pulmonary artery (PA) stenosis presents in different locations and may be congenital or occur after surgical intervention. Tetralogy of Fallot repair, BTS placement, arterial switch, or right ventricular to PA conduit placement for truncus arteriosus repair or pulmonary atresia may all lead to branch PA stenosis at the suture lines. Many of these sites become technically difficult to repair surgically and can be effectively treated in the catheterization laboratory with balloon angioplasty or more recently, with stent placement.

Balloon angioplasty of branch PA stenosis has a variable success rate. Approximately 60% of procedures are technically successful, but midterm follow-up suggests that up to two thirds have important residual stenosis.[32,33] This has led some interventionalists to treat branch PA stenosis with primary stent placement.[34] The implantable stent is a mesh of stainless steel that is tightened onto a balloon catheter and then advanced through a long sheath to the site of stenosis. The sheath is withdrawn and the balloon is inflated to dilate the stenosis. This expands the stent to the size of the balloon, and the radial strength of the stent prevents elastic recoil or refolding of the stenotic site. Multiple stents can be placed sequentially in long-segment stenosis. Bilateral stents can be placed at the same time with the "kissing" technique, which involves simultaneous stent implantation at the site of both proximal right and left PA stenoses (Fig 1). This prevents either stent from being partially collapsed or distorted by the inflation of a balloon in the contralateral PA.

Patients that require a surgical procedure and have distal pulmonary stenosis can also be treated with PA stenting in the operating room. The sites of the stenosis need to be well established before the surgical repair. The surgical field allows relatively easy access to the central PAs. A stent can then be advanced into the

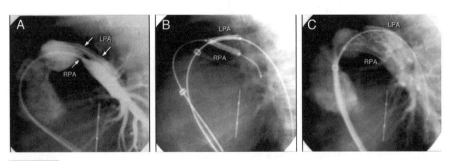

FIGURE 1.
Branch pulmonary artery *(PA)* stenosis: the "kissing" technique. A 5-month-old, 6-kg patient with truncus arteriosus repaired with a right ventricular to PA conduit. **A,** Severe proximal right PA *(RPA)* stenosis and left PA *(LPA)* stenosis marked with *arrows.* **B,** Balloon catheters with stents in proper position in both PAs just before simultaneous inflation. **C,** Stents in proper position with relief of the stenosis.

more distal PA under direct vision and palpation. When the surgeon and the cardiologist agree on proper position, the stent is implanted by inflating the balloon catheter. This technique is useful for patients who have failed attempts at stent placement in the catheterization laboratory or for patients without suitable venous access. A staged procedure with the stent placed before or after surgical repair is the more common therapy and is the preferred course.

The stents are available in a variety of sizes that can be redilated as the patients grow. The results of stent placement have been impressive with up to a 97% success rate. The complication rate is 2%.[34-36] Some of the concerns of placement of stents in smaller children include the need for a large introducing sheath, difficulty in placing a large enough stent, and the need for repeat catheterization to expand the stents as the child grows. The lifelong results of stent placement will continue to be evaluated as the patients reach adulthood. New stent technology will undoubtedly improve the results and allow smaller catheters and sheaths to be used. Future directions include self-expanding nitinol stents that can enlarge with the patient's growth, and absorbable stent material. Absorbable stents should obviate the need for large stent placement in small children and the potential difficulties a stainless steel stent could present at the time of subsequent surgical procedures.

Balloon angioplasty and stent placement have also been used to relieve stenosis within right ventricular to PA conduits. This can increase the interval between conduit replacement and possibly decrease the total number of sternotomies a patient requires. This is an important consideration for the best staged approach to complicated right ventricular outflow tract abnormalities.

COARCTATION ANGIOPLASTY

There is important controversy concerning the use of balloon angioplasty for native coarctation. The procedure has a success rate of approximately 80%, with success defined as a postprocedural gradient of less than 20 mm Hg.[37] There have been reports of up to a 20% incidence of aneurysm formation[38] and some incidence of restenosis.

The restenosis rate in neonates treated with balloon angioplasty is high (77%-83%). The restenosis is amenable to redilation, and the initial procedure can be lifesaving. This makes balloon angioplasty a reasonable interim therapy for situations when surgical repair is not possible. Balloon angioplasty has been used successfully for premature infants weighing as little as 460 g by using the umbilical artery, and also is used for abdominal coarctation.[39,40] The restenosis rate is reported to be much less in older children (7.3%-8%).[41,42] Long-term follow-up of adolescents and adults demonstrated normalization of blood pressure in 74% of patients treated with balloon angioplasty.[43] The reasonable success rate and low complication rate has led some groups to use balloon angioplasty as a primary treatment of choice for coarctation in adolescents and children outside of infancy.

We currently consider angioplasty for treatment of coarctations with gradients greater than 20 mm Hg in patients older than 1 year. Adolescents or adults with gradients between 10 and 20 mm Hg are considered for angioplasty with or without stent placement. This is done to decrease the long-term detrimental effects believed to result from these smaller degrees of obstruction and the increased obstruction present during exercise.

RECOARCTATION

The use of balloon angioplasty for recoarctation after surgical repair is less controversial, with early success rates of 88% to 91% and a restenosis rate of 16% to 28%.[44-46] Most cardiology–cardiothoracic surgery groups now use balloon dilation as the first-line therapy for postoperative recoarctation.

COARCTATION STENT

The need to dilate the coarctation segment to a size larger than the final anticipated diameter requires a large balloon and is thought to contribute to the risk of aneurysmal formation and the rare cases of fatal vessel rupture. Some groups have begun intervening at gradients of 10 to 15 mm Hg to reduce the long-term potential of hypertension and limit the known transient increase in gradient and hypertension that occurs with exercise. These goals and the limitation of the risks of angioplasty are easier to achieve with the use of intravascular stents and angioplasty for coarctation (Fig 2). The stent is enlarged to the measured size of the adjacent aorta with a balloon no larger in diameter than the transverse or descending aorta. This commonly results in a measured gradient of 0 to 10 mm Hg during the procedure and a predictable vessel diameter.[47,48] The stents can be further dilated in patients who still have growth potential. It is obviously important to place a stent that can be dilated to the size of an adult aorta to prevent future physiologic narrowing of the stented site. This limits the use of this tech-

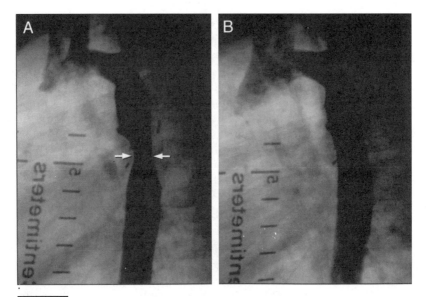

FIGURE 2.

Recoarctation stent. A 3½-year-old male child who had a patch angio-plasty repair of coarctation in infancy. **A,** Recoarctation at patch site *(arrows).* **B,** After stent placement with a Johnson & Johnson P-308 stent inflated with a 12-mm balloon, with no residual gradient.

nique to older children and adults. This technique has also been used for coarctations that were not effectively treated with balloon angioplasty alone, including long-segment coarctation.

Future technological developments with improved catheter and stent design and the potential for absorbable stents may increase the effectiveness of balloon angioplasty. This is an area of much active research and growing international experience with new equipment. The development of "covered stents," which are stents that have a nonpermeable membrane fixed circumferentially around the stent, is being investigated for the treatment of aneurysms.

Transcatheter intervention certainly complements the surgical repair of aortic arch abnormalities and has even been used to treat coarctation after the Norwood-type repair for hypoplastic left heart syndrome.[49] The treatment of coarctation must be tailored to each patient's anatomical abnormality and associated heart disease. Balloon angioplasty and the use of stents should be considered as a potential part of the treatment plan in any patient with coarctation.

PULMONARY VENOUS STENOSIS

Pulmonary venous stenosis is a rare but often lethal form of CHD with universally dismal results for surgical enlargement. Attempts at balloon dilation have produced immediate improvements in angiographic size, but restenosis of all dilated vessels occurs.[50] Stent placement in a stenotic pulmonary vein is also possible, with relief of stenosis. However, stent placement has not produced sustained improvement, as restenosis is the rule. Transcatheter interventions in the pulmonary veins are limited to transient palliation of patients who are awaiting more definitive surgical therapy, such as lung transplantation.

SYSTEMIC VEINS AND VENOUS CHANNELS

The success of the Senning and Mustard-type venous switches for the treatment of transposition of the great arteries has led to the long-term survival of many of these patients. A number of these patients have been noted to have progressive obstruction of their venous baffles. The surgical results of repair were not favorable, and transcatheter therapy with balloon dilation and stenting of the narrowed baffles was investigated.[51-52] Complete obstructions could be recanalized and residual gradients of zero were achieved with single or multiple stents. Redilation for neointimal hyperplasia–induced stenosis is also successful.[53] These same techniques can be applied for patients with Fontan circulation obstruction. Transcatheter stenting should be the intervention of choice for obstruction in venous vessels or channels.

OCCLUSION DEVICES

The use of devices for occlusion of PDA, ASD, ventricular septal defect (VSD), patent foramen ovale (PFO), and other vascular structures is the most rapidly advancing aspect of pediatric interventional catheterization. Multiple occlusion devices are currently available or under investigational trials.

VASCULAR OCCLUSION/EMBOLIZATION

Multiple substances have been used for occlusion/embolization of unwanted vascular structures since Portsmann's initial PDA occlusion. The current standard is Gianturco coils, which are small coiled spring wires with fabric strands woven into the springs. They are straightened and pushed through a small-diameter catheter to the site of occlusion. When extruded from the catheter they assume a coiled shape and induce thrombosis, which is promoted by the fabric strands. They are universally available in an array of sizes and are inexpensive.

Coils are useful for the occlusion of most abnormal collateral vessels. These are often found in patients with an abnormal pulmonary arterial supply and patients who have been palliated with Glenn shunts or have completed Fontan circulation for single ventricle physiology. The use of coil occlusion simplifies subsequent surgical procedures on these patients because it prevents the need for extensive surgical dissection to locate and ligate these vessels. The staged repair for these patients almost always requires a cardiac catheterization before surgical intervention, during which efforts to occlude any unnecessary collateral vessels should be attempted. The occlusion of collateral vessels can greatly reduce the pulmonary venous return and subsequent blood loss during bypass and allow an easier surgical procedure. There is also evidence that if collaterals are left without occlusion, pleural drainage after a Fontan completion may be prolonged.[54] Coils have been used for other purposes including occlusion of coronary-cameral artery fistulas, BTS, and pulmonary arteriovenous fistulas. Collateral occlusion should be considered a part of the routine care of these complex patients.[55-57]

Coils require a site of narrowing in the vessel to be occluded to prevent migration of the coil and are limited to structures less than 7 to 8 mm in diameter. This limitation led to the development of the Gianturco-Grifka vascular occlusion device (Cook Inc, Bloomington, Ind), a fabric sack into which a long coil is extruded that conforms to the size and shape of the vascular structure. Other devices have been used for occlusion of these same vessels, including the Amplatzer Duct Occluder and the Rashkind Occluder.

PATENT DUCTUS ARTERIOSUS

Efforts to perfect a transcatheter method for PDA occlusion have been ongoing since Portsmann et al[58,59] placed the first Ivalon foam plug prosthesis in 1967. Coil occlusion is currently the most commonly used technique. Coils are available as standard 0.035-, 0.038-, and 0.052-inch Gianturco coils (Cook Inc, Bloomington, Ind). The accurate placement of coils can be technically difficult, and multiple alternative delivery techniques have been devised to improve the success rate.

Devices have also been developed and evaluated to allow closure of larger PDAs and improved control of delivery. The Rashkind occluder and the buttoned device can be used for a variety of PDA sizes and types, but a significant incidence of initial residual shunts present at 1-year follow-up and risks of left PA stenosis have prevented their widespread acceptance.[60,61]

The Amplatzer Duct occluder (ADO) device was designed exclusively for PDA occlusion and, in the initial report, has proven to have excellent success, with a complete closure rate of 100% at 1-month follow-up and no complications.[62] The ADO device has several advantages over other available methods of PDA closure. It has a complete closure rate that is as high or is achieved sooner than other methods and has not been noted to have recurrence of shunting. It can be used effectively in cases of large PDAs up to 11 mm and can be used in all PDA types. The ADO can also be used in adults, in whom calcification of the PDA may be present and can complicate surgical closure.

These transcatheter techniques for PDA occlusion should be explored for patients with a simple PDA and can certainly be useful for patients with a contraindication to surgical closure of a PDA.

The ADO device has also been used successfully for closure of large coronary arteriovenous fistulas.[63] We have personal experience using the ADO device for occlusion of coronary artery fistulas, unnecessary BTSs, and pulmonary arteriovenous fistulas. The ADO device can be implanted in the efferent or afferent vessels in pulmonary arteriovenous fistulas, and successful occlusion can be achieved. We believe the ADO device is the most promising vascular occlusion device and can be useful for occlusion of any unwanted vascular connection.

ATRIAL SEPTAL DEFECT

Numerous devices have been developed and tested for ASD closure. There are several devices currently under investigation.

The first clamshell device has been modified since its early use and now has 2 versions, the CardioSEAL device and the self-centering version, the STARFlex Occluder (Nitinol Medical Technologies, Boston, Mass). The CardioSEAL device is expected to achieve at least the same results as its predecessor, the clamshell occluder, with 57% of patients having complete closure and 97% having complete closure or insignificant residual shunts at a mean follow-up of 41 months.[64] The STARFlex Occluder has not had a large series published. The button device has gone through 4 generations since its introduction in 1989. Results of phase 1 Food and Drug Administration trials demonstrated a complete closure rate of 74%, and 98% of 46 patients had at most a small residual shunt.[65] These excellent results have not been reproduced in international reports.[66,67] The Angel Wings device had a reported 96%

closure rate in 72 patients after 1 to 17 months of follow-up. This excellent closure rate was tempered by a 4% rate of serious complications and a device placement rate of only 71%.[68]

The most promising technique is ASD closure with the Amplatzer Septal Occluder (ASO) (AGA, Medical Corp, Golden Valley, Minn). The ASO device has a user-friendly delivery system, a high complete closure rate, a small delivery system to allow use in children, and the ability to retrieve or reposition the device before release from the delivery system.

The ASO device is a self-expanding double-disk device made from Nitinol wires, with Dacron polyester patches sewn into each disk and the connecting waist to increase the thrombogenicity of the device. The mechanism of closure involves stenting of the ASD by the waist of the device and subsequent thrombus formation within the device, with eventual complete neoendothelialization. To ensure stenting, a variety of device sizes are necessary.

The initial human use was reported in 1997, with correct placement in all 30 patients studied. Three-month follow-up was completed in 25 patients, and the complete closure rate was 100%.[69] Since that initial report, there have been multiple reports of initial experiences from investigators throughout the world.[70-74] The summary data from more than 1390 patients with devices implanted worldwide demonstrates an implantation rate of 95.6%, a complete closure rate of 91.26%, and a total success rate of 98.91% at 1 month, with success being defined as complete closure or at most the presence of a small residual shunt. These closure rates are high and compare favorably with those for surgical series.[75,76] Less than 1% of patients who had attempted closure required removal of an implanted device and surgical ASD closure. There have been no procedural-related deaths, and only 0.78% of patients had a serious complication. This low complication rate also compares favorably with that for surgical closure.[77,78] Some complications that have been associated with other devices have not been reported with the ASO device, specifically, wire fracture, late embolization, thromboembolic events, atrial perforation, pericardial effusion, and endocarditis.

The excellent initial experience with the ASO has led to its use in more complex cases and for other indications not related to ASD closure.[79,82] The ASO has finished phase 1 and 2 clinical trials in the United States, and the results have been very good.[83] The device is available outside of the United States for general use and is considered the first-line therapy for ASD closure in most institutions.[84]

The ASO device has demonstrated excellent clinical success in the closure of moderate-to-large secundum ASDs (Fig 3). The clo-

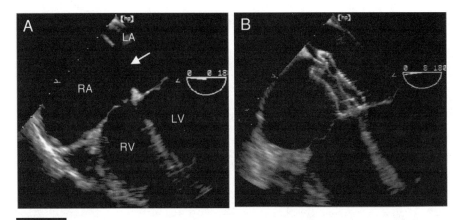

FIGURE 3.
Atrial septal defect (ASD) occlusion with the Amplatzer Septal Occluder. **A,** Transesophageal echocardiographic 4-chamber view demonstrating a 33-mm secundum ASD *(arrow)*. **B,** After device placement (38-mm Amplatzer Septal Occluder) with complete occlusion of the ASD. *Abbreviations: RA,* Right atrium; *LA,* left atrium; *RV,* right ventricle; *LV,* left ventricle.

sure rate is greater than 98%, and the implantation rate of 95.6% is exceptional. The ASO device is poised to be the procedure of choice for most secundum ASDs.

These ASD occlusion devices should be considered as possible primary therapy for secundum ASD occlusion and may be used in conjunction with surgical repair of CHD that does not require bypass. Contraindications to transcatheter ASD occlusion include associated CHD requiring cardiac surgery, partial anomalous pulmonary venous return, pulmonary vascular resistance greater than 7 Woods units, right-to-left shunting at the atrial level with a systemic saturation of less than 94%, recent myocardial infarction, unstable angina, decompensated congestive heart failure, or significant right or left ventricular decompensation with an ejection fraction of less than 30%.

FONTAN FENESTRATION

The fenestrated Fontan procedure was developed for patients to decrease the risk of morbidity and mortality after a Fontan completion. This procedure represents a perfect example of the potential collaborative efforts of congenital heart surgeons and interventional pediatric cardiologists. The surgical fenestration was created in the Fontan baffle with the intent to subsequently perform transcatheter closure of the fenestration. The increasing experience with transcatheter occlusion techniques has allowed multiple devices to be used for fenestration occlusion.

The original work with the Rashkind and clamshell occluders[85,86] has continued with the STARflex and CardioSEAL devices. The buttoned device was modified into an inverted buttoned device for use in fenestration occlusion.[87] The ASO has also been successfully used for fenestration occlusion.[88] Gianturco coils and detachable coils can also be effective for fenestration occlusion.[89,90] The technical consideration of coil occlusion has even prompted some surgeons to adapt their surgical procedure to create a fenestration that is more amenable to coil occlusion.[91] This certainly represents an ongoing staged approach to the management of single ventricle physiology that requires the talents of both congenital heart surgeons and interventionalists.

PATENT FORAMEN OVALE

The same devices that have been used for ASD closure have been used for PFO closure. Patients with a history of paradoxical embolism have been treated with either anticoagulation or surgical closure of their PFO. The introduction of transcatheter PFO closure has created a third option that prevents the risk of paradoxical embolism without the trauma of surgery or the risk of bleeding present with anticoagulation. The need for complete occlusion is much higher for this group of patients because any residual shunt may allow further embolism. The same rationale exists for avid scuba divers with a history of neurologic decompression illness.[92]

Transcatheter techniques are also possible for PFO closure in patients with the rare syndrome of Orthodeoxia-Platypnea, which consists of desaturation caused by a right-to-left shunt across a PFO that increases with upright posture. This debilitating condition is usually seen in patients with significant comorbidity that makes them high-risk surgical candidates. Transcatheter closure of the PFO and elimination of the right-to-left shunt produces immediate clinical improvement and should be considered the treatment of choice.

The Amplatzer PFO occluder has been designed exclusively for transcatheter occlusion of PFOs and is beginning clinical trials. The device is similar in construction to the ASO. The right atrial disk is larger than the left atrial disk and measures 25 or 35 mm. There is a short 3-mm waist segment. The initial results have been encouraging and have shown 100% successful placement and 100% complete occlusion. Long-term results and clinical follow-up are needed before transcatheter occlusion can be recommended for all patients with PFO and paradoxical embolism.

VENTRICULAR SEPTAL DEFECT

Many of the occlusion devices used for other shunts have also been used for VSD closure. Gianturco coils have been used to close small VSDs.[93,94] The Grifka bag has been used to close both muscular and perimembranous defects. The Rashkind devices have the longest record of VSD occlusion, with the ASD and PDA device both being used for VSD closure. Perimembranous, muscular, and postinfarction VSDs have all been effectively treated.[95-100]

The buttoned device has also been used for VSD closure, with 18 of 25 patients having devices placed in a multi-institutional study. Patients with membranous and muscular defects were selected for occlusion. Two devices needed to be surgically removed, and 13 of the remaining 16 patients had complete occlusion achieved.[101]

The Amplatzer VSD occluder device was designed exclusively for VSD closure and has been undergoing clinical trials since 1998. This device is designed for muscular VSD closure and can be effectively repositioned or retrieved until it is released in an optimal position. The device has been used for anterior, posterior, midmuscular, apical, postinfarction, and multiple "Swiss cheese"–type VSDs and has shown good results.[102-106] The long-term effects on ventricular dynamics and the cardiac conduction system have yet to be determined.

The preferred technique for all devices is transcatheter placement through percutaneous access, which avoids a surgical procedure and allows angiographic localization of the defect to be closed. The devices are often placed from a jugular approach, which allows a straight catheter course into the right ventricle and across the VSD. This is a relatively technically complex procedure that requires general anesthesia and is assisted by transesophageal echocardiographic guidance. A collaborative approach with device closure of a VSD during an open surgical procedure has also been performed with effective VSD occlusion.[107-109] This approach may improve device placement because the surgeon can position the device under direct vision, which could improve the successful implantation rate. We recently treated a patient with a large muscular VSD in whom the device, which was placed in the catheterization laboratory, was pushed partially into the left ventricle by the moderator band after release. The device was easily pulled back into the proper position and secured with a single suture through a small right ventriculotomy (Fig 4). It may be pos-

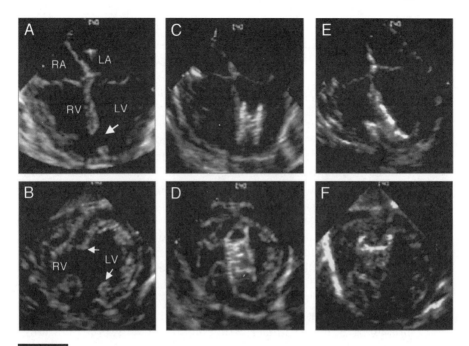

FIGURE 4.

Ventricular septal defect (VSD) occlusion with the Amplatzer Muscular VSD Occluder in a 4-month-old, 4.6-kg infant with large apical muscular VSDs and intractable heart failure. Transesophageal 4-chamber and short-axis echocardiographic images. **A,** Large muscular/apical VSD *(arrow).* **B,** Demonstration of the LV borders of the defect *(arrows).* **C** and **D,** Device location after release at catheterization. Note that the superior edge of the device has protruded into the LV chamber while the inferior edge straddles the septum appropriately. **E** and **F,** Device location after intraoperative repositioning of device into correct position and single-suture placement to fix the device on the septum. This was done through a small right ventriculotomy. *Abbreviations: RA,* Right atrium; *LA,* left atrium; *RV,* right ventricle; *LV,* left ventricle.

sible to avoid bypass and a large ventriculotomy by performing transcatheter device placement through a right ventricular puncture as performed in animal studies with the Amplatzer VSD occluder.[110]

The development of devices suitable for VSD closure has created an alternative to, and an adjunct treatment that can be used in conjunction with surgical VSD repair. Patients with complex CHD who require a staged approach to repair and patients with contraindications to surgical closure of their VSD have formed the early patient population undergoing transcatheter VSD occlusion. If the results of larger series of transcatheter VSD occlusion are comparable to the surgical results, this technique may become more widespread.

SUMMARY

The advances in pediatric interventional cardiac catheterization have changed the therapeutic strategy for many patients with CHD. The procedure of choice for valvar stenosis, recoarctation, collateral vessel occlusion, and branch PA stenosis has moved from the operating room to the catheterization laboratory. Effective and safe transcatheter interventions now exist for closure of ASDs, VSDs, and PDAs and are considered viable alternatives to surgical closure. Other interventional catheterization procedures are currently being investigated to complement the surgical management of patients with complex anatomy, including covered stents for repair of aortic aneurysms, covered stents to complete the Fontan circulation in patients after a modified Glenn shunt, multiple stent designs for all vascular stenoses, percutaneous PA band, and transcatheter resurrection of the pulmonary valve in patients with severe pulmonary regurgitation. The rapid advances in the technology used in the catheterization laboratory will serve to improve the care we provide for our patients and extend the range of interventions performed outside of the operating room.

Pediatric cardiologists and congenital heart surgeons must understand each other's interventional techniques and how they can be used in a coordinated fashion. This may involve staged therapy with transcatheter intervention before surgery, transcatheter interventions in the operating room, or modifications of surgical techniques to facilitate future interventional catheterization completion of a staged repair of complex disease. This interaction is essential for the optimal management of our patients with both straightforward lesions and complex anatomy.

ACKNOWLEDGMENT

We thank Dr Qi-Ling Cao for his assistance in preparing the figures for this chapter.

REFERENCES

1. Rashkind WJ, Miller WW: Creation of an atrial septal defect without thoracotomy: A palliative approach to transposition of the great arteries. *JAMA* 196:991-992, 1966.
2. Jamjureeruk V, Sangtawesin C, Layangool T: Balloon atrial septostomy under two-dimensional echocardiographic control: A new outlook. *Pediatr Cardiol* 18:197-200, 1997.

3. O' Laughlin MP, Mullins CE: Therapeutic cardiac catheterization, in Garson A Jr, Bricker JT, Fisher DJ, et al (eds): *The Science and Practice of Pediatric Cardiology.* Baltimore, Md, Williams & Wilkins, 1998, pp 2415-2419.

4. Park SC, Zuberbuhler JR, Neches WH, et al: A new atrial septostomy technique. *Cathet Cardiovasc Diagn* 1:195-201, 1975.

5. Park SC, Neches WH, Mullins CE, et al: Blade atrioseptostomy: Collaborative study. *Circulation* 66:258-266, 1982.

6. Kerstein D, Levy PS, Hsu DT, et al: Blade balloon atrial septostomy in patients with severe primary pulmonary hypertension. *Circulation* 91:2028-2035, 1995.

7. Seib PM, Faulkner SC, Erickson CC, et al: Blade and balloon atrial septostomy for left heart decompression in patients with severe ventricular dysfunction on extracorporeal membrane oxygenation. *Cathet Cardiovasc Intervent* 46:179-186, 1999.

8. Kan JS, White RI Jr, Mitchell SE, et al: Percutaneous balloon valvuloplasty: A new method for treating congenital pulmonary valve stenosis. *N Engl J Med* 307:540-542, 1982.

9. Lip GY, Singh SP, de Giovanni J: Percutaneous balloon valvuloplasty for congenital pulmonary valve stenosis in adults. *Clin Cardiol* 22:733-737, 1999.

10. Jarrar M, Betbout F, Farhat MB, et al: Long-term invasive and noninvasive results of percutaneous balloon pulmonary valvuloplasty in children, adolescents, and adults. *Am Heart J* 138:950-954, 1999.

11. Stanger P, Cassidy SC, Girod DA, et al: Balloon pulmonary valvuloplasty: Results of the Valvuloplasty and Angioplasty of Congenital Anomalies Registry. *Am J Cardiol* 65:775-783, 1990.

12. Colli AM, Perry SB, Lock JE, et al: Balloon dilation of critical valvar pulmonary stenosis in the first month of life. *Cathet Cardiovasc Diagn* 34:23-28, 1995.

13. Wang JK, Wu MH, Lee WL, et al: Balloon dilation for critical pulmonary stenosis. *Int J Cardiol* 69:27-32, 1999.

14. Gildein HP, Kleinert S, Goh TH, et al: Treatment of critical pulmonary valve stenosis by balloon dilatation in the neonate. *Am Heart J* 131:1007-1011, 1996.

15. Siblini G, Rao PS, Singh GK, et al: Transcatheter management of neonates with pulmonary atresia and intact ventricular septum. *Cathet Cardiovasc Diagn* 42:395-402, 1997.

16. Hijazi ZM, Patel H, Cao QL, et al: Transcatheter retrograde radio-frequency perforation of the pulmonic valve in pulmonary atresia with intact ventricular septum, using a 2 French catheter. *Cathet Cardiovasc Diagn* 45:151-154, 1998.

17. Akagi T, Hashino K, Maeno Y, et al: Balloon dilatation of the pulmonary valve in a patient with pulmonary atresia and intact ventricular septum using a commercially available radio-frequency catheter. *Pediatr Cardiol* 18:61-63, 1997.

18. Gibbs JL, Blackburn ME, Uzun O, et al: Laser valvotomy with balloon

valvuloplasty for pulmonary atresia with intact ventricular septum: Five years' experience. *Heart* 77:225-228, 1997.

19. Justo RN, Nykanen DG, Williams WG, et al: Transcatheter perforation of the right ventricular outflow tract as initial therapy for pulmonary valve atresia and intact ventricular septum in the newborn. *Cathet Cardiovasc Diagn* 40:408-413, 1997.

20. Wang JK, Wu MH, Chang CI, et al: Outcomes of transcatheter valvotomy in patients with pulmonary atresia and intact ventricular septum. *Am J Cardiol* 84:1055-1060, 1999.

21. Cheatham JP: The transcatheter management of the neonate and infant with pulmonary atresia and intact ventricular septum. *J Intervent Cardiol* 11:363-387, 1998.

22. Leung MP, Lo RN, Cheung H, et al: Balloon valvuloplasty after pulmonary valvotomy for babies with pulmonary atresia and intact ventricular septum. *Ann Thorac Surg* 53:864-870, 1992.

23. Ovaert C, Qureshi SA, Rosenthal E, et al: Growth of the right ventricle after successful transcatheter pulmonary valvotomy in neonates and infants with pulmonary atresia and intact ventricular septum. *J Thorac Cardiovasc Surg* 115:1055-1062, 1998.

24. Labadidi Z, Wu RJ, Walls TJ: Percutaneous balloon aortic valvuloplasty: Results in 23 patients. *Am J Cardiol* 53:194-197, 1984.

25. Sholler GF, Keane JF, Perry SB, et al: Balloon dilation of congenital aortic stenosis: Results and influence of technical and morphological features on outcome. *Circulation* 78:351-360, 1988.

26. Fischer DR, Ettedgui JA, Park SC, et al: Carotid artery approach for balloon dilation of aortic valve stenosis in the neonate: A preliminary report. *J Am Coll Cardiol* 15:1633-1636, 1990.

27. Weber HS, Mart CR, Kupferschmid J, et al: Transcarotid balloon valvuloplasty with continuous transesophageal guidance for neonatal critical aortic valve stenosis: An alternative to surgical palliation. *Pediatr Cardiol* 19:212-217, 1998.

28. Neish SR, O' Laughflin MP, Nihill MR, et al: Intraoperative balloon valvuloplasty for critical aortic valvular stenosis in neonates. *Am J Cardiol* 68:807-810, 1991.

29. Brown JW, Robison RJ, Waller BF: Transventricular balloon catheter aortic valvotomy in neonates. *Ann Thorac Surg* 39:376-378, 1985.

30. Kuhn MA, Latson LA, Cheatham JP, et al: Management of pediatric patients with isolated valvar aortic stenosis by balloon aortic valvuloplasty. *Cathet Cardiovasc Diagn* 39:55-61, 1996.

31. Rao PS: Balloon aortic valvuloplasty. *J Intervent Cardiol* 11:319-329, 1998.

32. Kan JS, Marvin WJ Jr, Bass JL, et al: Balloon angioplasty—branch pulmonary artery stenosis: Results from the Valvuloplasty and Angioplasty of Congenital Anomalies Registry. *Am J Cardiol* 65:798-801, 1990.

33. Ettinger LM, Hijazi ZM, Geggel RL, et al: Peripheral pulmonary artery stenosis: Acute and mid-term results of high pressure balloon angioplasty. *J Intervent Cardiol* 11:337-344, 1998.

34. Formigari R, Casado J, Santororo G, et al: Treatment of peripheral pulmonic stenoses. *J Intervent Cardiol* 11:331-336, 1998.
35. O' Laughlin MP, Slack MC, Grifka RG, et al: Implantation and intermediate-term follow-up of stents in congenital heart disease. *Circulation* 88:605-614, 1993.
36. Hijazi ZM, Al-Fadley F, Geggel RL, et al: Stent implantation for relief of pulmonary artery stenosis: Immediate and short-term results. *Cathet Cardiovasc Diagn* 38:16-23, 1996.
37. McCrindle BW, Jones TK, Morrow WR, et al: Acute results of balloon angioplasty of native coarctation versus recurrent aortic obstruction are equivalent. For the Valvuloplasty and Angioplasty of Congenital Anomalies (VACA) Registry Investigators. *J Am Coll Cardiol* 28:1810-1817, 1996.
38. Shaddy RE, Boucek MM, Sturtevant JE, et al: Comparison of angioplasty and surgery for unoperated coarctation of the aorta. *Circulation* 87:793-799, 1993.
39. Schamberger MS, Lababidi ZA: Successful balloon angioplasty of a coarctation in an infant <500 g. *Pediatr Cardiol* 19:418-419, 1998.
40. Adwani S, De Giovanni JV: Percutaneous transluminal balloon angioplasty of abdominal coarctation in an infant. *Pediatr Cardiol* 17:346-348, 1996.
41. Fletcher SE, Nihill MR, Grifka RG, et al: Balloon angioplasty of native coarctation of the aorta: Midterm follow-up and prognostic factors. *J Am Coll Cardiol* 25:730-734, 1995.
42. Rao PS, Galal O, Smith PA, et al: Five to nine-year follow-up results of balloon angioplasty of native coarctations in infants and children. *J Am Coll Cardiol* 27:462-470, 1996.
43. Fawzy ME, Sivanandum V, Pieters F, et al: Long-term effects of balloon angioplasty on systemic hypertension in adolescents and adults with coarctation of the aorta. *Eur Heart J* 20:827-832, 1999.
44. Yetman AT, Nykanen D, McCrindle BW, et al: Balloon angioplasty of recurrent coarctation: A 12-year review. *J Am Coll Cardiol* 30:811-816, 1997.
45. Hijazi ZM, Geggel RL: Balloon angioplasty for postoperative recurrent coarctation of the aorta. *J Intervent Cardiol* 8:509-516, 1995.
46. Mahechwari S, Bruckheimer E, Fahey JT, et al: Balloon angioplasty of postsurgical recoarctation in infants: The risk of restenosis and long-term follow-up. *J Am Coll Cardiol* 35:209-213, 2000.
47. Harrison DA, McLaughflin PR: Interventional cardiology for the adult patient with congenital heart disease: The Toronto Hospital experience. *Can J Cardiol* 12:965-971, 1996.
48. Ebeid MR, Prieto LR, Latson LA: Use of balloon-expandable stents for coarctation of the aorta: Initial and intermediate-term follow-up. *J Am Coll Cardiol* 30:1847-1852, 1997.
49. Zellers TM: Balloon angioplasty for recurrent coarctation of the aorta in patients following staged palliation for hypoplastic left heart syndrome. *Am J Cardiol* 84:231-233, 1999.

50. Driscoll DJ, Hesslein PS, Mullins CE: Congenital stenosis of individual pulmonary veins: Clinical spectrum and unsuccessful treatment by transvenous balloon dilatation. *Am J Cardiol* 49:1767-1772, 1982.

51. Chatelain P, Meier B, Friedli B: Stenting of superior vena cava and inferior vena cava for sympathetic narrowing after repeated atrial surgery for D-transposition of the great vessels. *Br Heart J* 66:466-468, 1991.

52. Ward CJB, Mullins CE, Nihill MR, et al: Use of intravascular stents in systemic venous and pulmonary venous baffle obstructions. Short-term follow-up results. *Circulation* 91:2948-2954, 1995.

53. Trerosola SO, Lund GB, Samphilipo MA, et al: Palmaz stent in the treatment of central venous stenosis: Safety and efficacy of redilation. *Radiology* 190:379-385, 1994.

54. Spicer RL, Uzark KC, Moore JW, et al: Aortopulmonary collateral vessels and prolonged pleural effusions after modified Fontan procedures. *Am Heart J* 131:1164-1168, 1996.

55. Kanter KR, Vincent RN, Raviele AA: Importance of acquired systemic–to-pulmonary collaterals in the Fontan operation. *Ann Thorac Surg* 68:969-974, 1999.

56. Perry SB, Radtke W, Fellows KE, et al: Coil embolization to occlude aortopulmonary collateral vessels and shunts in patients with congenital heart disease.

57. Furman BP, Bass JL, Casteneda-Zuniga W, et al: Coil embolization of congenital thoracic vascular anomalies in infants and children. *Circulation* 70:285-289, 1984.

58. Portsmann W, Wierny L, Warnke H: Der Verschluss des Ductus arteriosus persistens ohne Thorakotamine (1, Miffeilung). *Thoraxchirurgie* 15:109-203, 1967.

59. Portsmann W, Wierny L, Warnke H: Catheter closure of patent ductus arteriosus: 62 cases treated without thoracotomy. *Radiol Clin North Am* 9:203-218, 1971.

60. Dessy H, Hermus JPS, van den Heuvel F, et al: Echocardiographic and radionuclide pulmonary blood flow patterns after transcatheter closure of patent ductus arteriosus. *Circulation* 94:126-129, 1996.

61. Rao PS, Sideris EB: Transcatheter occlusion of patent ductus arteriosus: State of the art. *J Invas Cardiol* 8:278-288, 1996.

62. Masura J, Walsh KP, Thanopoulous B, et al: Catheter closure of moderate- to large-sized patent ductus arteriosus using the new Amplatzer duct occluder: Immediate and short-term results. *J Am Coll Cardiol* 31:878-882, 1998.

63. Thomson L, Webster M, Wilson N: Transcatheter closure of a large coronary artery fistula with the Amplatzer duct occluder. *Cathet Cardiovasc Intervent* 48:188-190, 1999.

64. Prieto LR, Foreman CK, Cheatham JP, et al: Intermediate-term outcome of transcatheter secundum atrial septal defect closure using the Bard clamshell septal umbrella. *Am J Cardiol* 78:1310-1312, 1996.

65. Zamora R, Rao PS, Lloyd TR, et al: Intermediate-term results of

phase I food and drug administration trials of buttoned device occlusion of secundum atrial septal defects. *J Am Coll Cardiol* 31:674-676, 1998.

66. Lambert V, Losay J, Piot JD, et al: Late complications of percutaneous closure of atrial septal defects with the Sideris occluder. *Arch Mal Coeur Vaiss* 90:245-251, 1997.

67. Arora R, Trehan VK, Kalra GS, et al: Transcatheter closure of atrial septal defect using buttoned device: Indian experience. *Indian Heart J* 48:145-149, 1996.

68. Rickers C, Hamm C, Stern H, et al: Percutaneous closure of secundum atrial septal defect with a new self-centering device (angel wings). *Heart* 80:517-521, 1998.

69. Masura J, Gavora P, Formanek A, et al: Transcatheter closure of secundum atrial septal defects using the new self-centering Amplatzer septal occluder: Initial human experience. *Cathet Cardiavasc Diagn* 42:388-393, 1997.

70. Thanopoulos BD, Laskari CL, Tsaousis GS, et al: Closure of atrial septal defects with the Amplatzer occlusion device: Preliminary results. *J Am Coll Cardiol* 31:1110-1116, 1998.

71. Chan KC, Godman MJ, Walsh K, et al: Transcatheter closure of atrial septal defect and interatrial communications with a new self-expanding nitinol double disc device (Amplatzer septal occluder): Multicenter UK experience. *Heart* 82:300-306, 1999.

72. Wilkinson JL, Goh TH: Early clinical experience with the use of the 'Amplatzer septal occluder' device for atrial septal defect. *Cardiol Young* 8:295-302, 1998.

73. Berger F, Ewert P, Bjornstad PG, et al: Transcatheter closure as standard treatment for most interatrial defects: Experience in 200 patients treated with the Amplatzer septal occluder. *Cardiol Young* 9:468-473, 1999.

74. Dhillon R, Thanopoulos B, Tsaousis G, et al: Transcatheter closure of atrial septal defects in adults with the Amplatzer septal occluder. *Heart* 82:559-562, 1999.

75. Pastorek JS, Allen HD, Davis JT: Current outcomes of surgical closure of secundum atrial septal defect. *Am J Cardiol* 74:75-77, 1994.

76. Meijboom F, Hess J, Szatmari A, et al: Long-term follow-up (9-20 years) after surgical closure of atrial septal defect at a young age. *Am J Cardiol* 72:1431-1434, 1993.

77. Pastorek JS, Allen HD, Davis JT: Current outcomes of surgical closure of secundum atrial septal defect. *Am J Cardiol* 74:75-77, 1994.

78. Berger F, Vogel M, Alexi-Meskishvili V, et al: Comparison of results and complications of surgical and Amplatzer device closure of atrial septal defects. *J Thorac Cardiovasc Surg* 118:674-678, 1999.

79. Hakim F, Madani A, Samara Y, et al: Transcatheter closure of secundum atrial septal defect in a patient with dextrocardia using the Amplatzer septal occluder. *Cathet Cardiavasc Diagn* 43:291-294, 1998.

80. Pedra CAC, Fontes-Pedra SRF, Esteves CA, et al: Multiple atrial septal defects and patent ductus arteriosus: Successful outcome using two

Amplatzer septal occluders and Gianturco Coils. *Cathet Cardiavasc Diagn* 45:257-25, 1998.

81. Hope SA, Partridge J, Slavik Z: A novel use of an Amplatzer septal occluder. *Heart* 81:672-673, 1999.

82. Tofeig M, Walsh KP, Arnold R: Transcatheter occlusion of a post-Fontan residual hepatic vein to pulmonary venous atrium communication using the Amplatzer septal occluder. *Heart* 79:624-626, 1998.

83. Hijazi ZM, Radtke W, Ebeid MR, et al: Transcatheter closure of atrial septal defects using the Amplatzer septal occluder: Results of phase II US multicenter trial (abstract). *Circulation* 100:I-804S, 1999.

84. Berger F, Ewert P, Bjornstad PG, et al: Transcatheter closure as standard treatment for most interatrial defects: Experience in 200 patients treated with the Amplatzer septal occluder. *Cardiol Young* 9:468-473, 1999.

85. Bridges ND, Lock JE, Castaneda AR: Baffle fenestration with subsequent transcatheter closure. Modification of the Fontan operation for patients at increased risk. *Circulation* 82:1681-1689, 1990.

86. Bridges ND, Casteneda AR: The fenestrated Fontan procedure. *Herz* 17:242-245, 1992.

87. Rao PS, Chandar JS, Sideris EB: Role of inverted buttoned device in transcatheter occlusion of atrial septal defects or patent foramen ovale with right-to-left shunting associated with previously operated complex cardiac anomalies. *Am J Cardiol* 80:914-921, 1997.

88. Tofeig M, Walsh KP, Chan C, et al: Occlusion of Fontan fenestrations using the Amplatzer septal occluder. *Heart* 79:368-370, 1998.

89. Sommer RJ, Recto M, Golinko RJ, et al: Transcatheter coil occlusion of surgical fenestration after Fontan operation. *Circulation* 94:249-252, 1996.

90. Gamillscheg A, Beitzke A, Stein JI, et al: Transcatheter coil occlusion of residual interatrial communications after Fontan procedure. *Heart* 80:49-53, 1998.

91. Sanatani S, Sett SS, Human DG, et al: Extracardiac Fontan operation with tube fenestration allowing transcatheter coil occlusion. *Ann Thorac Surg* 66:933-934, 1998.

92. Walsh KP, Wilshurst PT, Moarrison WL: Transcatheter closure of patent foramen ovale using the Amplatzer septal occluder to prevent recurrence of neurological decompression illness in divers. *Heart* 81:257-261, 1999.

93. Latiff HA, Alwi M, Kandhavel G, et al: Transcatheter closure of multiple muscular ventricular septal defects using Gianturco coils. *Ann Thorac Surg* 68:1400-1401, 1999.

94. Kalra GS, Verma PK, Dhall A, et al: Transcatheter device closure of ventricular septal defects: Immediate results and intermediate-term follow-up. *Am Heart J* 138:339-344, 1999.

95. O' Laughlin MP, Mullins CE: Transcatheter occlusion of ventricular septal defect. *Cathet Cardiovasc Diagn* 17:175-179, 1989.

96. Rigby ML, Redington AN: Primary transcatheter umbrella closure of

perimembranous ventricular septal defect. *Br Heart J* 72:368-371, 1994.

97. Janorkar S, Goh T, Wilkinson J: Transcatheter closure of ventricular septal defects using the Rashkind device: Initial experience. *Cathet Cardiovasc Intervent* 46:43-48, 1999.

98. Benton JP, Barker KS: Transcatheter closure of ventricular septal defect: A nonsurgical approach to the care of the patient with acute ventricular septal rupture. *Heart Lung* 21:356-364, 1992.

99. Lock JE, Block PC, McKay RG, et al: Transcatheter closure of ventricular septal defects. *Circulation* 78:361-368, 1988.

100. Bridges ND, Perry SB, Keane JF, et al: Preoperative transcatheter closure of congenital muscular ventricular septal defects. *N Engl J Med* 324:1312-1317, 1991.

101. Sideris EB, Walsh KP, Haddad JL, et al: Occlusion of congenital ventricular septal defects by the buttoned device. "Buttoned device" Clinical Trials International Register. *Heart* 77:276-279, 1997.

102. Thanopoulos BD, Tsaoisis GS, Konstadopoulou GN, et al: Transcatheter closure of muscular ventricular septal defects with the Amplatzer ventricular septal defect occluder: Initial clinical applications in children. *J Am Coll Cardiol* 33:1395-1399, 1999.

103. Hijazi ZM, Hakim F, Al-Fadley, et al: Transcatheter closure of single muscular ventricular septal defects using the Amplatzer ventricular septal defect occluder: Initial results and technical considerations. *Cathet Cardiovasc Intervent* 49:167-172, 2000.

104. Tofeig M, Patel RG, Walsh KP: Transcatheter closure of a mid-muscular ventricular septal defect with an Amplatzer VSD occluder. *Heart* 81:438-440, 1999.

105. Lee EM, Roberts DH, Walsh KP: Transcatheter closure of a residual postmyocardial infarction ventricular septal defect with the Amplatzer septal occluder. *Heart* 80:522-524, 1998.

106. Rodes J, Piechaud JF, Ouakine R, et al: Transcatheter closure of apical ventricular septal defect combined with arterial switch operation in a newborn infant. *Cathet Cardiovasc Intervent* 49:173-176, 2000.

107. Murzi B, Bonanomi GL, Giusti S, et al: Surgical closure of muscular ventricular septal defects using double umbrella devices (intraoperative VSD device closure). *Eur J Cardiothorac Surg* 12:450-454, 1997.

108. Chaturvedi RR, Shore DF, Yacoub M, et al: Intraoperative apical ventricular septal defect closure using a modified Rashkind double umbrella. *Heart* 76:367-369, 1996.

109. Fishberger SB, Bridges ND, Keane JF, et al: Intraoperative device closure of ventricular septal defects. *Circulation* 88:205-209, 1993.

110. Amin Z, Gu X, Berry JM, et al: Periventricular closure of ventricular septal defects without cardiopulmonary bypass. *Ann Thorac Surg* 68:149-153, 1999.

CHAPTER 9

Turbine Blood Pumps

George P. Noon, MD
Professor of Surgery, Michael E. DeBakey Department of Surgery; Chief, Division of Transplant and Assist Devices, Baylor College of Medicine; Executive Director, Multi-organ Transplant Center, The Methodist Hospital, Houston, Tex

Deborah Morley, PhD
Vice President, Clinical Affairs, MicroMed Technology, Inc, Houston, Tex

Suellen Irwin, RN
Research Associate, Michael E. DeBakey Department of Surgery, Baylor College of Medicine, Houston, Tex

Sandy Abdelsayed
Manager, Clinical Affairs, MicroMed Technology, Inc, Houston, Tex

Robert Benkowski, BSME
Vice President, Engineering, MicroMed Technology, Inc, Houston, Tex

Bryan E. Lynch, BSME, MBA
Director of Operations, MicroMed Technology, Inc, Houston, Tex

Nearly 5 million people in the United States today are affected by congestive heart failure, with more than 400,000 new patients being diagnosed each year. Heart failure affects people of all ages, and, since the aging population is the most commonly affected, the number of people with heart failure will grow over the next few decades.[1] At present, options for treatment of end-stage heart failure include medical management and, for a limited group of patients, cardiac transplantation. Should medical therapy fail for the transplant candidate, a variety of ventricular-assist devices and artificial hearts are available for use as bridges to transplantation. In view of the increasing population with heart failure, there is a need to develop long-term cardiac-assist devices that are effective, safe, and simple to operate, that allow unrestricted mobility, and that are economically feasible.

A variety of pulsatile and nonpulsatile cardiac-assist devices are available or are being developed for circulatory assistance. Devices are applied most commonly for cardiopulmonary resuscitation, surgical procedures, failure to wean from cardiopulmonary bypass after cardiotomy, extracorporeal membrane oxygenation (ECMO), bridging to transplantation, bridging to recovery, and permanent support. Device selection depends on the patient's condition and size, as well as on the type and duration of support required. Most systems used for short-term support (ie, several weeks), such as the roller or centrifugal pump, are continuous-flow pumps. When desired, pulsatility can be enhanced if systems are combined with the intra-aortic balloon pump. Most clinical and laboratory research has shown that pulsatility in short-term support has some advantages over nonpulsatile flow in blood distribution, systemic vascular resistance, organ and tissue perfusion, and cellular metabolism.[2,3] Despite these observations, however, systems with limited or no pulsatility are successfully and predominantly used in short-term support.

The development of devices for long-term or permanent support has focused primarily on pulsatile ventricular-assist devices and artificial hearts. These devices have proved successful in providing both short- and long-term circulatory support. The success of the support depends on the occurrence of device-related complications and the condition of the patient when support is initiated. For the next generation of devices, there has been increasing interest in developing a continuous-flow pump for long-term patient support. A continuous-flow pump may offer many advantages over the pulsatile devices. Such a design is smaller; is easier to implant; has less surface in contact with blood; requires no valves, air vent, or compliance chamber; uses less power; has fewer moving parts; makes less noise; and could be more durable and less expensive. A smaller pump could fit in smaller patients and would require less dissection to implant. Clearly, continuous-flow assist devices have some configuration advantages.[4] The question is: Will the blood flow that they provide be sufficient to support the patients and their circulatory needs?

In normal human circulation, the arteries transport blood pumped from the heart, under high pulsatile pressure, to the arterioles. Arterioles act as control valves for blood flow into the capillaries. Pulsatility is dissipated at the capillary level, where fluid, nutrients, electrolytes, hormones, and other substances are exchanged between the blood and the interstitial fluid. Venules collect blood from the capillaries, and blood flows into the larger veins and then back to the right side of the heart. As the blood is transported through the arterial system, the normal pulsatile blood pressures in the aorta are 120 mm Hg during systole and 80 mm Hg during diastole. Blood pressure decreases as blood circulates through the arterioles, capillaries, and the venous system and diminishes to nearly 0 mm Hg at the termination of the venae cavae in the right atrium.

Pressures in capillaries near the arterioles average 35 mm Hg, and pressures in capillaries near the venous end average as low as 10 mm Hg. In general, the functional pressure of the vascular bed averages 17 mm Hg. In the pulmonary circulation, there is a pulsatile pressure averaging 16 mm Hg in the arteries, becoming lower or nonpulsatile on the venous side. Many other factors influence the regulation of circulation to meet the needs of the tissues. Among these additional control mechanisms are baroreceptors, neuroendocrine factors, and endothelial substances. In summary, blood pressure and pulsatility decrease as blood flows through both the systemic and pulmonary circulatory systems. Seventy percent of the blood flow is normally nonpulsatile in the vascular system.[5]

If pulsatility is nearly absent in the capillaries, where tissues are nourished and wastes are removed, is pulsatility in the arterial system an absolute requirement for human survival? Can nonpulsatile flow in the arterial system maintain a satisfactory blood flow and arterial-venous pressure gradient? Blood flow through a vessel is determined by the difference in pressure between the 2 ends of the vessel and the vascular resistance. Ohm's Law describes how flow is calculated: Blood flow equals the pressure difference between the 2 ends of the vessel divided by the resistance. Rate of flow is determined by the pressure differential between the two ends of the vessel, not the absolute pressure in the vessel.[5] Of note, the velocity of transmission of the pressure pulse is 15 or more times the velocity of blood flow in the aorta. Pressure pulse is a moving wave of pressure with very little forward movement of blood volume.[6] Clinical and experimental studies have shown that nonpulsatile flow can maintain adequate pressures, flows, and resistance, thereby providing adequate hemodynamics for survival.[3,7]

THE MICROMED DEBAKEY VENTRICULAR-ASSIST DEVICE

In 1988, a team of researchers from the Baylor College of Medicine, led by Drs George Noon and Michael DeBakey, met with engineers from the National Aeronautics and Space Administration's (NASA's) Johnson Space Center. They began a comprehensive research process to develop a miniature axial blood-flow pump, to be used as a ventricular-assist device (VAD)in patients with end-stage heart failure. MicroMed Technology, Inc (Houston, Texas) received the license for the technology in June 1996 and since has been developing the MicroMed DeBakey VAD for commercial use.[4,8,9]

DESIGN RATIONALE

The objective of the designers was to develop a VAD system that was safe, effective, reliable, user-friendly, and affordable. The design of the axial flow pump was targeted to reduce hemolysis, thrombosis, noise, and heat generation. Design specifications included an implantable axial flow pump that could pump at least 5 L/min against 100-mm Hg pressure. The goal for the entire system was to allow patients to move about freely with a portable controller and battery. With this type of design, the recipient might recover from the effects of heart failure, be discharged from the hospital, perform the normal activities of daily living, and have a better quality of life.[4,8,9]

PRECLINICAL TESTING

Preclinical testing of the MicroMed DeBakey VAD was divided into several phases, each of which had a specific objective. During the first phase of studies, a polycarbonate version of the pump was used. The purpose was to develop a pump design that resulted in the least possible hemolysis and thrombosis. The least-hemolytic design was identified through parametric bench testing of several design iterations. Next, ex vivo tests of iterative pump designs were conducted to identify the pump that was least thrombogenic. For these tests, a polycarbonate pump was mounted in a saddle on a calf's back so that blood flowed through the device until thrombosis occurred or the experiment duration was met. This model was used to finalize a pump design that could be used for up to 2 weeks without significant hemolysis or thrombosis.

The next group of studies was performed in vivo; that is, a titanium pump was implanted intrathoracically in 24 calves. The purpose was to verify with the titanium pump that the least hemolytic and least thrombogenic design had been identified. The study also determined the safety of the MicroMed DeBakey VAD for long-term support. The MicroMed DeBakey VAD was shown to operate safely in animals for up to 145 days. Average pump outputs were maintained above 3.0 L/min with power consumption of 10 W or less. No significant hemolysis or end-organ dysfunction occurred. Complications included 1 case of device-related infection and 2 cases of pump thrombus. One of the cases of pump thrombus occurred after a malfunction in an early controller model. The second case involved a small hub thrombus. These experiments allowed for final design of the external components of the system, the controller and the Clinical Data Acquisition System (CDAS).

Further in vivo studies were conducted to assess the safety of the entire system (pump, controller, CDAS) in support of European clinical trials. Six of the 8 calves studied in this phase of preclinical testing survived 90 days after implantation. One animal was killed soon after surgery because its hypercontractile ventricle obstructed flow through the pump. Another animal was killed because of a pump stoppage on day 24 after implantation. Explant analyses showed a ring thrombus at the rear bearing. Pump output for the 6 surviving animals ranged from 3.3 to 5.4 L/min. Power consumption was 10 W or less. There was no end-organ dysfunction, hemolysis, or infection. Although minor mechanical malfunctions did occur, such as the freezing of a computer screen and the disconnection of a cable, each was readily resolved. Occasional episodes of resynchronization (momentary stop and restart) were noted; however, in all cases the pump restarted according to design. The results supported the safety of the entire system's configuration, and European clinical trials began in November 1998.

In vitro performance tests have been conducted with mock circulation, to define characteristics of pump function in response to normal and abnormal vascular conditions and ventricular performance. Completed studies to date show that the MicroMed DeBakey VAD can unload the failing left ventricle adequately and perform as expected when physiological parameters such as preload or heart rate are varied.

Other studies are ongoing to determine whether "bearing wear" can be detected vibroacoustically. Two types of studies are being conducted: induced wear and endurance tests. The objective of induced-wear tests is to quantify the relationship between artificially induced bearing wear, hemolysis, and the resulting vibroacoustic signature. No significant level of hemolysis has been observed at any level of artificially induced bearing wear, and no difference in hemolysis has been shown between any artificially induced bearing-wear steps. The objective of the endurance tests is to examine endurance and assess bearing wear during continuous pump operation. As part of the endurance tests, 10 pumps operated continuously for up to 30 months. Only 2 pumps showed evidence of minimal wear.

Implantable components of the MicroMed DeBakey VAD system have been subjected to both hemocompatibility and biocompatibility studies. The purpose of hemocompatibility studies was to identify blood-titanium interactions with the MicroMed DeBakey VAD. These tests were performed with human blood in mock circulation. The pump was not a source for either thrombi or emboli and was otherwise hemocompatible. Biocompatibility tests were negative with respect to systemic toxicity, local toxicity, cytotoxicity, genotoxicity, pyrogenicity, physiochemical toxins, mutagenicity, and sensitization. The process by which implantable components are sterilized in ethylene oxide also was validated.

Design controls consistent with the requirements outlined by the Quality Systems Regulation of the US Food and Drug Administration(21 CFR 820), the International Organization for Standardization (ISO) 9000 guidelines, European Norm (EN) 46001, and the European Active Implantable Medical Device Directive (AIMDD) (90/385/EEC) were used in the development of the pump, controller, and data-acquisition system. Over 50 pump-design iterations were evaluated by NASA design engineers. The controller and CDAS systems were designed by subcontractors who had ISO 9001 certification. MicroMed Technology, Inc assembles the subsystems and distributes the final system.[8]

DESCRIPTION AND HUMAN CONFIGURATION OF FINAL PUMP DESIGN

The MicroMed DeBakey VAD system meets the design goals by providing a system that allows the recipient to move about freely with a portable controller and batteries. Fig 1 depicts the MicroMed DeBakey VAD human configuration and final pump design. The MicroMed DeBakey VAD system consists of 4 subsystems: a pump system (Fig 2, Fig 3), a controller system (Fig 4), a CDAS (Fig 5), and a Patient Home Support System (PHSS)(Fig 6).

PUMP SYSTEM

The titanium, electromagnetically actuated axial flow pump can pump in excess of 10 L/min, is 1.2 in (30.5 mm) in diameter, is 3.0 in (76.2 mm) long, and weighs 95 g. The priming volume of the pump, including the inflow cannula, is 25 mL. The pump system consists of a titanium inflow cannula and apical ring, the MicroMed DeBakey VAD pump, a flow probe, a Dacron outflow conduit graft, and a percutaneous cable assembly with controller connector (Fig 3).

Inside the housing unit is the impeller/inducer, which is the only moving part. Connected to the flow tube is a curved titanium

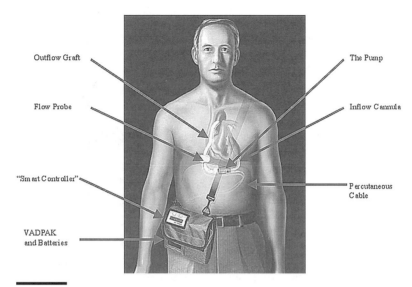

FIGURE 1.
The MicroMed DeBakey VAD human configuration. Components of the system are labeled by the *arrows.* Note the mobility this configuration allows the patient.

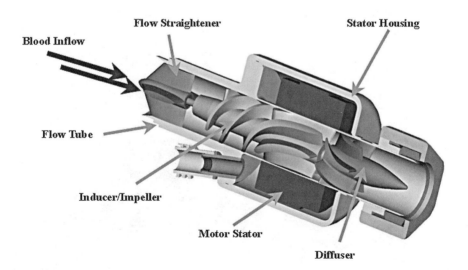

FIGURE 2.
The MicroMed DeBakey VAD pump components.

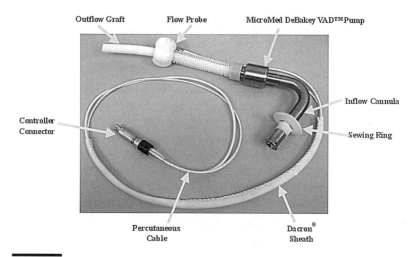

FIGURE 3.
Assembled MicroMed DeBakey VAD pump.

inflow cannula that is inserted into the left ventricular apex and secured to an apical ring sewn to the left ventricle. A Dacron-sealed, woven outflow conduit is connected to the pump and sewn to the ascending aorta. An ultrasonic flow probe placed around the outflow conduit continually measures blood flow rate through the pump. The wiring from the pump's flow probe and motor are coated and bundled into a single cable assembly covered by Dacron

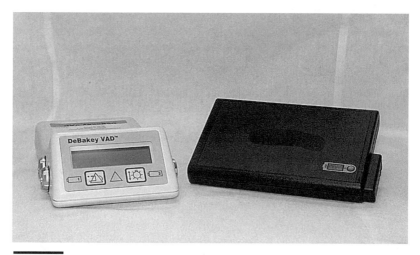

FIGURE 4.
MicroMed DeBakey VAD Controller and Battery.

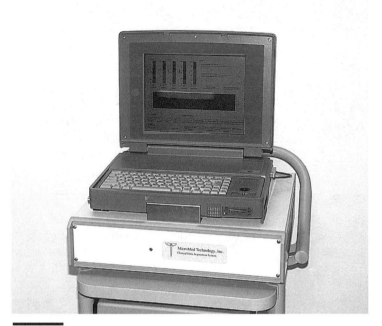

FIGURE 5.
Clinical Data Acquisition System (CDAS).

velour, which exits the skin from the abdominal wall superior to the right iliac crest and connects to the external controller system. Blood flows from the left ventricular inflow cannula into the flow tube, out through the outflow conduit, and into the ascending aorta (Fig 1). This axial flow pump provides continuous flow. Depending on the strength of the heart's native contractility and the resulting difference in pressure (ΔP) between the left ventricle and aorta, however, flow pulsatility does exist.[4,8,9]

CONTROLLER SYSTEM

The controller is designed to operate the pump system. It is completely external and consists of the controller module, battery packs, and a battery charger. The 4 × 6-in controller module has audible and visual alarms with messages and prompts displayed on the controller module's scrollable liquid-crystal display (LCD) (Fig 4). Two intelligent battery packs can be connected to the controller module to power the pump, or the controller can be connected to the CDAS for power.

The VAD system is designed for simple operation by both the recipient and the clinician. During the development of the pump system, a VADPAK (Fig 1) was designed to provide the recipient with a safe, ergonomic, small, and comfortable external transport mechanism.[4,8,9]

CLINICAL DATA ACQUISITION SYSTEM

The CDAS is a laptop-based system that stores pump-operating data, displays pump and physiological information, and is used by clinicians to modify the pump speed (Fig 5). It also serves as a primary power source for the pump and is used to stop and start the pump during surgery.[4,8,9]

PATIENT HOME SUPPORT SYSTEM

The PHSS (Fig 6) is a small unit that serves as a battery charger and provides wall power to the controller when the patient is at home or in the regular ward of the hospital. It also serves as an emergency battery back-up for the patient at home in the event of a power outage.

INDICATIONS

The MicroMed DeBakey VAD currently is indicated for use as a bridge to heart transplantation in patients who have been accept-

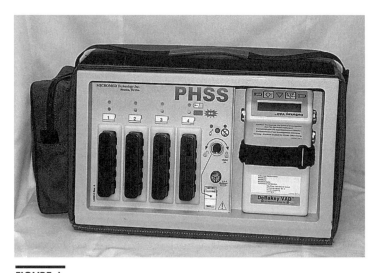

FIGURE 6.
The Patient Home Support System (PHSS). Four batteries can be charged with the small unit, which also stores a spare controller for the patient.

ed by an institution's transplant committee but who have not yet received the device implant. Future indications for the MicroMed DeBakey VAD may be as a bridge to recovery and as a chronic implant. The small size of the VAD is advantageous in that it can be implanted in smaller patients compared with the pulsatile VADs and requires less operative dissection. Use of the MicroMed DeBakey VAD extracorporeally in small children and infants is another potential application.[4,8]

PATIENT SELECTION

Patients with advanced heart failure who were transplant candidates and whose condition was rapidly deteriorating underwent implantation in the clinical trial of the MicroMed DeBakey VAD. In general, to qualify for the study, patients must have been transplant candidates and shown profound cardiac failure. Cardiac failure could be confirmed either by hemodynamics (elevated pulmonary capillary wedge pressure, low cardiac index, etc.) or by the need for extraordinary inotropic support, including intra-aortic balloon counterpulsation. There were no exclusions to implantation, other than those that would typically exclude a patient from cardiac transplantation. The criteria used for the clinical trial were similar to those used during clinical investigations of left ventricular assist devices currently on the market. The MicroMed DeBakey VAD currently is used as a bridge to transplantation in patients with advanced heart failure. Future uses may include post-cardiotomy ventricular support, bridging to recovery, and permanent implantation.

IMPLANTATION TECHNIQUES

Patients with left ventricular failure requiring left ventricular assistance often are in the preliminary stages of multiorgan failure. In many patients, end-organ dysfunction will require multiorgan support during and immediately after implantation. A temporary right ventricular assist device should be available for patients who have right-sided heart failure after VAD implantation despite optimal medical management. A continuous vein-vein hemofiltration system may be necessary for patients with fluid overload due to excessive infusion of crystalloid or blood products during implantation. An intra-aortic balloon pump also should be available to provide hemodynamic support and counterpulsation when necessary. A transesophageal or transthoracic echocardiogram is valuable for evaluating bilateral ventricular function, the presence of a patent foramen ovale, and visualizing air or clotting in the left ventricle. Transesophageal echocardiography also should be used to evaluate the position of the inflow cannula in the left ventricle before closing the chest.

Before beginning the operation, the pump is immersed in a solution of dextrose 5% and water, connected to the controller, and tested. An outflow graft is mounted and secured to the outflow end of the pump. A flow probe is placed on the outflow graft to measure pump flows after implantation.

For pump implantation, a median sternotomy incision is performed extending several inches below the xiphoid process. A small abdominal-wall pocket is formed below the rectus muscle. The size and configuration of the pocket is determined by using the actual or mock pump as a model. To provide access to the left ventricular apex, the pericardium is opened, the diaphragmatic attachment to the costal margin is divided, and both are extended laterally beyond the apex. Meticulous hemostasis is important.

The patient is given heparin in preparation for cardiopulmonary bypass. A cannula is inserted into the ascending aorta, then 1 or 2 cannulas are inserted into the right atrium and cava, depending upon the presence of a patent foramen ovale. Cardiopulmonary bypass can begin when desired. If a patent foramen ovale is detected by echocardiogram or right atrial exploration, it is repaired before beginning the VAD implantation.

The left ventricular apex is elevated and the insertion site of the inflow cannula is selected. The apical fixation ring is sewn in place with at least 8 interrupted mattress sutures, using 2-0 polypropylene with large Teflon felt pledgets. A trocar is connected to the pump driveline to aid in tunneling of the cable from the abdominal-wall pocket across the midline to exit the skin in a convenient position above the right iliac crest. The trocar is then removed and the driveline is connected to the controller.

The left ventricular apex is elevated again to prepare for insertion of the pump's inflow cannula. The heart can be beating, fibrillating, or arrested. With use of a #11 blade, a full-thickness cruciate incision is made inside the apical ring. The ventricular apex is compressed manually to prevent bleeding. A round-bladed coring device is inserted into the left ventricle to extract a core of the left ventricular apex. The apical tissue is removed from the coring device and carefully examined for completeness to confirm precise apical coring and extraction. Digital ventricular exploration is performed to evaluate the position of the core and to ensure the absence of potential obstructions to inflow. Visual exploration of the ventricle may be necessary for further removal of myocardium or clot. The pump outflow graft is clamped, and the inflow cannula is inserted into the left ventricular apex.

Proper placement of the inflow cannula inside the ventricle is imperative. The goal is to place the inflow cannula so that it is angled toward the aortic valve without being directed toward the myocardial septum or free wall. The inflow-cannula position can be adjusted by moving the body of the pump in the pocket. The cannula opening must be clear of any ventricular tissue. By using the polypropylene sutures placed previously, the suture ring on the inflow cannula is sewn to the apical fixation ring. Air is removed from the pump and left ventricle by allowing the ventricle to fill with blood. The pump and outflow graft are elevated and filled with blood from the ventricle by releasing and reapplying the clamp on the outflow graft. The apical insertion site is carefully checked for bleeding. To ensure hemostasis, it may be necessary to further seal the ventricular sewing-ring attachment by approximating the left ventricular apex and the sewing ring with a Teflon felt strip and continuous 2-0 polypropylene sutures.

The MicroMed DeBakey VAD is placed into the abdominal pocket and the length of the outflow graft is measured and trimmed. The graft should lie under the right sternal border without kinking or overstretching. A proximal, external graft protector is designed to prevent graft kinking. Care is taken to ensure that the flow probe is placed immediately proximal to the graft protector, because this helps in proper positioning of the outflow graft. A partial-occlusion clamp is placed on the ascending aorta. A longitudinal arteriotomy is made, and the outflow graft is sewn to the lateral ascending aorta using 5-0 polypropylene. After completion of the anastomosis, an 18-gauge needle is placed in the outflow graft between the aortic anastomosis and the graft clamp. With temporary release of the clamp, the distal aortic graft is filled with blood, and trapped air escapes through the needle. The aorta is reclamped. Remaining air in the system is released through the 18-gauge needle by unclamping the outflow graft and intermittently starting and stopping the pump. The clamp is then removed, and continuous pumping is begun at 7500 rpm. After all remaining air is released, the 18-gauge needle is removed and a pledgeted 4-0 polypropylene suture is used to oversew the needle hole.

Pump flows are then adjusted to maintain a cardiac index of about 2.0 L/min/m^2 or greater. To maintain sufficient pump flow, it is important to ensure adequate preload. Hypovolemia and excessive pump speed could result in ventricular collapse and diminished flows. With use of echocardiography, the location of the inflow cannula is viewed and the ventricles are assessed for volume, function, and the presence of air. The inflow cannula must be free of obstruction. When placement of the cannula is considered satisfactory and flows are adequate, the patient is weaned from cardiopulmonary bypass and protamine is given to reverse the heparin. After meticulous hemostasis, drains are placed in the mediastinum and pump pocket and the incision is closed. The driveline exit site is approximated and the line is secured in place with a suture.[4,8]

POSTOPERATIVE CONSIDERATIONS

For optimal pump and cardiac function, it is important to maintain adequate preload, afterload, ventricular function, and cardiac rhythm. After surgery, inotropic medications are continued to support the right ventricle. Because of the continuous pumping action of the pump, some degree of inotropic support for the right ventricle should be maintained for at least 48 hours, to ensure that the right heart is ready to accept the increasing demand. If the right ventricle fails despite medical management, a temporary or long-term right ventricular-assist device is implemented. An intra-aortic balloon pump also may be inserted for temporary pulsatile flow or hemodynamic support if desired. After coagulopathies have been controlled and postoperative bleeding has been minimized, the patient is placed on anticoagulant therapy. This usually begins within 24 to 48 hours after implantation. The current recommendation for anticoagulation is to start the patient on intravenous heparin or subcutaneous low-molecular-weight heparin, then convert to warfarin, aspirin, and clopidogrel bisulfate.

Patients with a continuous-flow pump may not have palpable pulses or blood pressures audible with a sphygmomanometer. Because the pulse is diminished, pulse oximeters may not measure peripheral oxygen saturation accurately. Indwelling arterial catheters or a Doppler may be needed to evaluate blood flow and measure blood pressure in heart-failure patients with continuous-flow devices.[4,8]

MICROMED DEBAKEY VAD CLINICAL EXPERIENCE

The MicroMed DeBakey VAD was the first axial flow pump to undergo clinical trials. The first trial began in Europe in November 1998 and has enrolled 44 patients as of August 2000. Three additional patients have undergone implantation at the author's institution in Houston since June 2000, under an Investigational Device Exemption (IDE) protocol. Twelve of the 47 total patients (40 men,

7 women) have undergone successful cardiac transplantation. A detailed evaluation of the first 32 patients has been completed, for which statistics are presented here. Support duration has ranged up to 133 days; 21 patients have been supported for more than 30 days, and 13 patients have been supported for more than 60 days. The median time to transplantation has been 74.5 days with a median support duration of 47 days. The cumulative number of patient-days of support is 1876.

Fifty percent of the patients enrolled in the clinical trials had idiopathic dilated cardiomyopathies; 38% had ischemic cardiomyopathies. On study entry, the mean cardiac index was 1.7 L/min/m^2 with an average mean pulmonary artery pressure of 25 mm Hg. With current data, the probability of survival at 30 days after the MicroMed DeBakey VAD implant is 81%. Eleven of the 32 patients underwent cardiac transplantation, and 10 of the 32 patients died while on VAD support. Only one death had a potential relationship to the device. Most of the deaths occurred because of multiorgan failure in patients who were the sickest before implantation. These patients may not have recovered with any form of mechanical support.

Results of the European clinical trial clearly show that the MicroMed DeBakey VAD can provide adequate circulatory support in patients with severe heart failure. Fig 7 illustrates the

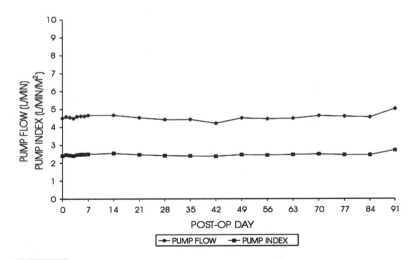

FIGURE 7.
Pump flow (L/min) and pump index (L/min/m^2) are illustrated. Pump flow remained above 4 L/min and pump index remained above 2.3 L/min/m^2, showing that all patients received adequate perfusion regardless of body size.

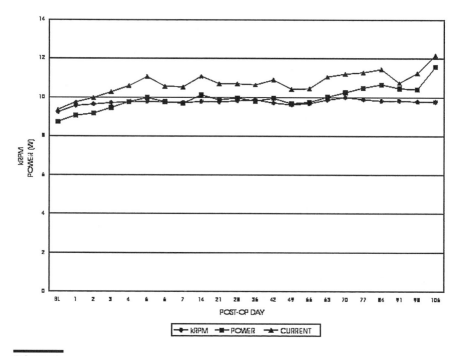

FIGURE 8.
Trends in speed (krpm), power (W) and current (A) for 90 days of MicroMed
DeBakey VAD support. There was little change in any of these variables over
time.

trends in total pump flow and pump index values over 90 days of
support. Pump flow ranged from 3.9 to 5.4 L/min. This flow was
adequate to meet perfusion needs of all patients, regardless of
size, as shown by the pump index values, which ranged from 2.5
to 2.8 L/min/m². Fig 8 illustrates the speed, power, and current
requirements for the device during this time and shows that adequate pump performance was maintained at relatively low energy
costs.

Our analysis of the first 32 patients on the MicroMed DeBakey
VAD support illustrates that end-organ function was either maintained or improved during the course of support. Fig 9 shows the
trends for measures of renal function (blood urea nitrogen [BUN]
and creatinine) and hepatic function (total bilirubin). Although
most patients who died had multiorgan failure, this could not be
related to device performance. There was no difference in pump
index values or flow pulsatility between survivors and nonsur-
vivors. Most of the patients who died of multiorgan failure had

perioperative intra-aortic balloon pumps that insured pulsatile flow.

The principal complication observed in the clinical trials has been late bleeding, with most events occurring more than 5 days after implantation surgery. This bleeding appears to be related to anticoagulation; after review of the data with investigators, reduction of the target International Normalized Ratio (INR) to 2.0 to 2.5 has reduced the incidence of bleeding. Some cases of hemolysis also have been observed. These events, all occurring more than 16 days after implantation, have been transient in some cases, and they have occurred at only 4 of the 10 institutions actively enrolling patients in the trial. No device-related infections have been observed, most likely because of the small size and flexibility of the percutaneous cable. One very minor cerebrovascular accident has occurred. All device events that have occurred have been minor, have been readily corrected, and have not jeopardized patient safety. A small number of patients have developed pump thrombus or embolus that affected pump function, which has required pump exchange or outflow-graft ligation to prevent regurgitant flow or continued support.

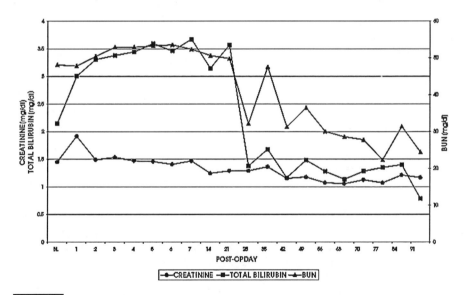

FIGURE 9.

Trends in BUN (mg/dL), creatinine (mg/dL), and total bilirubin (mg/dL) for 90 days of MicroMed DeBakey VAD support. End-organ function did not worsen significantly and may have improved, although later trends may be affected by sample size.

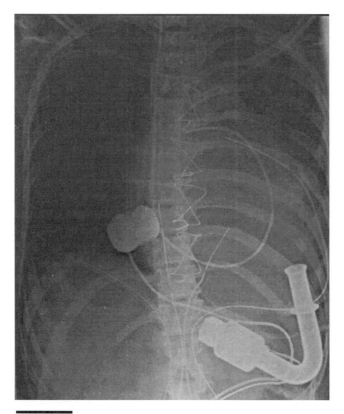

FIGURE 10.
Chest X ray from a 17-year-old patient who received the MicroMed DeBakey VAD. His body surface area was 1.54 m^2. The chest x-ray film shows how easily the device fits in smaller patients.

Many advantages of the MicroMed DeBakey VAD have been observed during the clinical trials. Investigators have found the ease and reduced time of surgical implantation to be desirable compared with other devices. Skin-to-skin times for implantation have been in the range of 2 to 3 hours, reducing patient exposure to anesthesia, cardiopulmonary bypass, and other complications of surgery. Only 2 of the 32 patients implanted have encountered significant perioperative bleeding. For this reason, investigators have selected the MicroMed DeBakey VAD over other available devices at their centers in cases where previous thoracic surgeries would increase the risk of surgical bleeding. Investigators have found that the miniature size of the MicroMed DeBakey VAD has allowed them to place the device in women or small-framed men, who otherwise would have required an extracorporeal device (Fig 10). Investigators participating in the European clinical trial have found postoperative management to be uncomplicated. Most patients have become mobile quickly after implantation. Several have participated in postimplantation bicycle ergometer training programs and have been able to achieve workloads of greater than 50 W without alteration of device settings. In several cases, patients have been able to spend weekends at home and make other out-of-hospital trips (Fig 11). One patient was at his home for nearly a month, awaiting cardiac transplantation, before a flu-like infection brought him back to the hospital.

CLINICAL HEMODYNAMICS

The MicroMed DeBakey VAD is a continuous, axial flow pump whose output is determined by the pump rpm and the difference in pressure (ΔP) between inflow and outflow. At a fixed rpm, pump output in patients will vary depending upon left ventricular pressure changes during the cardiac cycle and the central aortic pressure. Continuous flow produced by the pump may be steady or pulsatile depending upon the ΔP (Fig 12). Most supported patients showed some degree of pulsatile blood flow and pressure even when the aortic valve did not open.

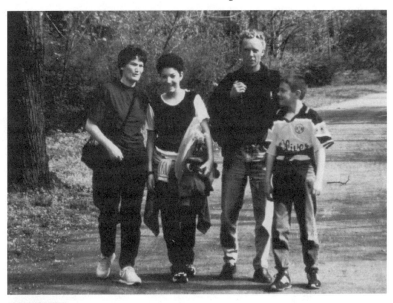

FIGURE 11.
A patient outside of the hospital walking with family.

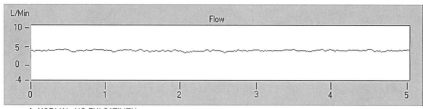

A. NORMAL NO PULSATILITY

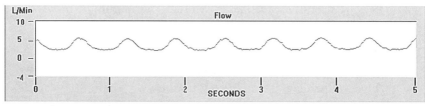

B. NORMAL MODERATE PULSATILITY

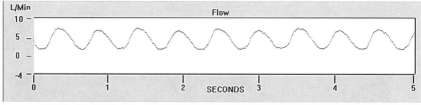

C. NORMAL PULSATILITY

FIGURE 12.
Examples of normal flow with the MicroMed DeBakey VAD. **A,** Normal; no pulsatility. **B,** Normal; moderate pulsatility. **C,** Normal; pulsatility.

Pump flow may decrease when the rpm increases above a certain level, resulting in progressive ventricular unloading and a decrease in ventricular pressure. This could result in partial or complete ventricular collapse (Fig 13). In this situation, the only way to improve flow is to reduce rpm and or increase the preload.

Most patients, when stable, have had the pump set at a fixed rpm that provides a pump index of 2.5 L/min/m^2. These patients were able to perform normal activities and exercise. An occasional patient has had a transient nocturnal decrease in flow.

FUTURE CONSIDERATIONS

A potential concern with continuous-flow devices is the possibility of regurgitant flow into the heart if the pump stops, which

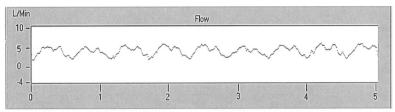

A. VENTRICULAR FUNCTION WITH SUCTION - PRODUCES ERRATIC WAVE FORM WITH MULTIPLE PEAKS

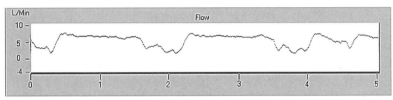

B. SUCTION WITH NO NATIVE VENTRICULAR FUNCTION

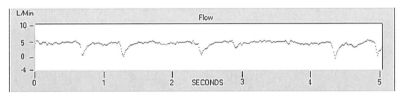

C. NO NATIVE VENTRICULAR FUNCTION SUCTION PRODUCES SHARP DOWNWARD GRADIENTS IN FLOW

FIGURE 13.
Examples of excess suction with the MicroMed DeBakey VAD. **A,** Ventricular function with suction; produces erratic waveform with multiple peaks. **B,** Suction with no native ventricular function. **C,** No native ventricular function; suction produces sharp downward gradients in flow.

could worsen the patient's heart failure. To address this possibility, a pump design is being considered that would prevent regurgitation by occluding the outflow graft.

At this time, the system does not incorporate an automatic speed control. The pump speed is fixed and can be changed only when the controller is attached to the CDAS. A situation could occur in which a patient would benefit from a change in pump speed, but this would be impossible because the patient is not connected to the CDAS. A planned future generation of the MicroMed

DeBakey VAD will include a controller that has an adjustable flow-rate algorithm, which will adapt pump flows to the patient's hemodynamic and metabolic needs.[4,8]

SUMMARY

After years of development and preclinical testing, clinical trials of the MicroMed DeBakey VAD began in November 1998 in Europe and in June 2000 in the United States. As of August 2000, 44 patients in Europe and 3 patients in the United States have undergone implantation with the MicroMed DeBakey VAD.

In conclusion, data from the European clinical trial of the MicroMed DeBakey VAD support the safety and performance of the device. Results show that the device provides adequate left ventricular and circulatory support in patients with end-stage heart failure without unduly jeopardizing patient safety. Moreover, the device provides advantages not inherent to commercially available pulsatile devices: (1) miniature size, enabling implantation in smaller patients; (2) ease of implantation; (3) reduced surgical bleeding; and (4) a low incidence of postoperative infections, often a limiting factor with other devices. The MicroMed DeBakey VAD European clinical trial is the first demonstration of the compatibility of continuous blood flow with adequate tissue perfusion and overall maintenance of life for up to 4.5 months. This initial experience with the MicroMed DeBakey VAD suggests that the pump can provide circulatory support to bridge patients to cardiac transplantation and may provide an improved quality of life for the patient with end-stage heart failure.

REFERENCES

1. American Heart Association: Living with Heart Failure, Information and Support for Patients and Caregivers. Available at http://www.americanheart.org/chf.
2. Hornick P, Taylor K: Pulsatile and nonpulsatile perfusion: the continuing controversy. *J Cardiothorac Vasc Anes* 11:310-315, 1997.
3. Jett GK: Physiology of nonpulsatile circulation: acute versus chronic support. *ASAIO J* 45:119-122, 1999.
4. Noon GP, Morley D, Irwin S, et al: Development and clinical application of the MicroMed DeBakey VAD. *Curr Opin Cardiol* 15:166-171, 2000.
5. Guyton AC: Overview of the circulation, and medical physics of pressure, flow, and resistance, in Wonsiewicz MJ, Hallowell R, Raymond J (eds): *Textbook of Medical Physiology*, 8th ed. Philadelphia, WB Saunders Co, 1991, pp 150-158.
6. Guyton AC: Vascular distensibility and functions of the arterial and

venous systems, in Wonsiewicz MJ, Hallowell R, Raymond J (eds): *Textbook of Medical Physiology*, 8th ed. Philadelphia, WB Saunders Co, 1991, pp 159-169.

7. Yozu R, Golding LA, Jacobs G, et al: Experimental results and future prospects for a nonpulsatile cardiac prosthesis. *World J Surg* 9:116-127, 1985.

8. Noon GP, Morley D, Irwin S, et al: The DeBakey ventricular assist device, in Goldstein DJ, Oz MC (eds): *Cardiac Assist Devices*. New York, Futura Publishing Co, 2000, pp 375-386.

9. Noon GP, Hetzer R, Loebe M, et al: Clinical experience with the DeBakey VAD axial flow pump. *Cardiovasc Eng* 5:30-32, 2000.

Index